Yoga
and
NUTRITION

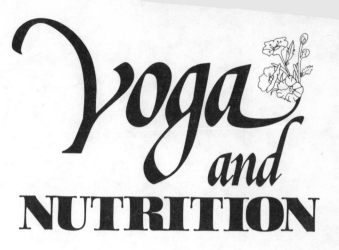

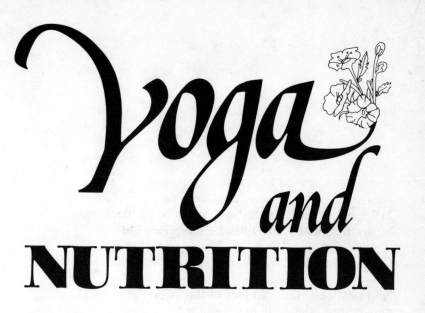

Yoga and NUTRITION

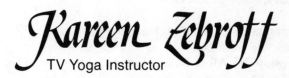

Kareen Zebroff

TV Yoga Instructor

ARCO PUBLISHING, INC.
219 PARK AVENUE SOUTH, NEW YORK, N.Y. 10003

Published 1979 by Arco Publishing, Inc.
219 Park Avenue South, New York, N.Y. 10003
by arrangement with Fforbez Enterprises Ltd.

Photographs by Duncan McDougall, Vancouver, B.C.

Cover photo by Alber Schoepflin, Frankfurt, West Germany

Edited by Kenneth D. McRae

Library of Congress Cataloging in Publication Data

Zebroff, Kareen.
  Yoga and nutrition.

  Bibliography: p. 184
  Includes index.
  1. Yoga, Hatha.   2. Nutrition.   I. Title.
RA781.7.Z44   613.7   78-13437
ISBN 0-668-04711-9

Printed in the United States of America

DEDICATION

To Peter and our daughters:
Sylvie, Tanya and Petra

ACKNOWLEDGEMENTS

I would like to express my special thanks to
Patricia Birkett for her most informative letters.

CONTENTS

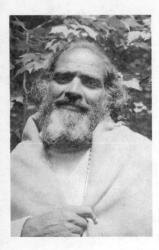

FOREWORD

by Swami Shyam Acharya

When I first met Kareen Zebroff she said "When the Chela (student) is ready, the Guru (teacher) appears." I immediately responded to this ancient traditional saying of Yoga teachers, "No, Kareen, when the Guru becomes ready or perfect, the student appears."

There are hundreds of teachers these days but no disciples because students are now born at that level of awareness which guides them easily to the teachers they need for their growth. This is not a time of blind faith or belief. If the teacher is not capable enough to project his wisdom, then none will be interested in learning from him. It appears then that, consciously or subconsciously, Kareen has been led by Creative Intelligence to become a perfect teacher and to create an opportunity for people to follow her instructions. She tuned her body to health, beauty, suppleness, and strength and then found her students coming to her through the medium of television.

The moment I met her I found her to be the best listener: calm, smiling, and easily comprehending. As a result, of the group with her she was the one to whom I spoke, though I had never seen her before. Such meetings I attribute to Almighty Creative Intelligence which is the guiding force for both student and teacher. That force I call the master teacher for it directs the consciousness of all the masters in the world.

In this foreword I have not to say too much about Kareen because she, through her teachings and books, is already known to nearly all aspirants of

Yoga across Canada. Her books and her lessons indicate by themselves the efficiency of her particular version of ancient India's secret wisdom—Yoga.

The West is very open and is not clouded by any secrecy as far as science is concerned. Western minds plunge to the depths and soar to the heights of every subject in which they are interested. I admire this tendency in any mind, eastern or western, because it is the key to obtaining knowledge. Unless one questions, doubts the reality of anything with which he is not familiar, how can he find the truth? Obviously, Kareen is typically western on this point. She has questioned the secrecy and vague intricacies of some presentations of Yoga. Not finding a scientific answer from those teachers who had introduced Yoga to the West with a negative attitude towards life such as don't eat this thing; renounce materiality; renounce the world and family; maintain celibacy; obey your teachers blindfoldedly, etc, she evolved and molded her own yoga.

Since time immemorial in the East, it was expected that the student never should question the master. He should accept whatever is said. But that is not the way in the West. Here one questions first and deserves the answer by his questioning. The time has come for a balance between dogmatism and open inquiry, secrecy and frankness. Such a balance is true Yoga.

Through constant practice and full devotion to her subject Kareen has made herself a symbol of health for her family and countrymen. One must certainly appreciate her desire to extend whatever she has gained to others. Several thousand years ago, Patangali, the father of yoga, said, "The true teacher is one who never teaches. Men receive his teachings as the world of darkness receives the light from the sun, without ceremony." Surely, this applies to Kareen.

There is one important point which I have always emphasized while talking and consulting with Kareen and others interested in yoga. It is not a study only of physical exercises. They are just one aspect of Yoga. We must know the true meaning of Yoga. Yoga is that state of life which in its perfect form holds the positive and negative qualities of everything in balance and never swings lower or higher from its yoked position. It remains ever established in harmony: serene, peaceful, full of joy, full of happiness and full of that cohesive material of God which connects the whole universe—Love. From my own experience with Yoga, I have found that it improves man in all his four aspects: physically, mentally, intellectually, and spiritually. Indeed, it not only improves him, I am confident that Yoga makes man perfect.

When Kareen heard me she said, "Well Swamiji, I have little to do with the teaching of the mental and spiritual sides of yoga, though I appreciate them very much myself. I needed the knowledge of them and you supplied it. But it is hard for the western mind to accept the non-physical side so I give emphasis to Hatha Yoga which I call Kareen's Yoga." Listening to her words I told her, "That is good. You have adopted just one aspect of yoga: Karma Yoga, the yoga of action." Now it so happens that her name, Kareen, coincides with a word from one of the Indian languages (Punjabi) which means "please do it". So Kareen's Yoga means "practical Yoga". This is easy, simple, scientific and can easily be adapted by western minds and I am sure, if she goes to the East, eastern women would like to do her way of yoga too.

As I have suggested, the thinking being needs exercise as well as the physical being. If the realms of the mind are not stirred and given the right experiences, no brain will develop adequately to grasp the realities of life, happiness and immortality, realities which Western man is in a craze to know. Therefore, I introduce the inner wisdom of Yoga which is entirely concerned with concentration, contemplation and meditation. Without them, no man, whatever his position in life, can become great. It is the need of modern man to become the highest and greatest of that which he is capable. Such a need can be satisfied through meditation and the technique of highest awareness (samadhi). If man learns this technique the world as a whole will experience an era of golden fulfillment, of joy, love and extreme tolerance for all life. That perfect state of mind is Yoga.

As far as meditation is concerned, I want to impress upon all minds, western or eastern, that meditation is a thinking process and not a chemical production of the plastic age. It concerns man alone and only the man of higher awareness. Therefore, meditation cannot be put on a par with sports, exercises, or with physical hatha yoga. Meditation concerns those who are desirous of improving their physical environments, family affairs, and the affairs vitally concerned with the welfare of mankind. To them I say that they should shift their attention from the outer aspect of life towards the inner man who wants to grow and fulfill himself at any cost, under any circumstances. Fathom the workings of the mind and when doing something channel your total energy into it. The source of energy must be handled in such a way that no wastage by way of scattered thoughts and confused thinking may take place.

How to grasp and practice the technique of samadhi may be a little hard for the reader to understand, but I will make it as simple as truth is simple. Create a situation of utter silence, rather super silence. You know already that "Silence is power, silence is golden," and we all know that we want power and gold.

More than immortality, we want to enjoy eternity. Here, every mind is my follower. Now, these things are not to be found without doing something. They must be earned. So for inner and outer power and gold, create a situation around you and in you of pure silence. Sleep doesn't produce silence because the nervous system doesn't completely rest. Lying in dead posture also does not provide this complete silence. The way to attain it is to sit comfortably in a chair or on the floor or in any corner no matter what noise is going on. Listen to anything. Think of anything. Above all, *be a Witness Self.* Watch and be. When your eyes and ears wish to take rest, please don't be cruel. Give them rest. Just be simple, no complications, no secrets, no religion.

Of course, as you become more familiar with this state of silence your understanding of it will grow. Above all, for growth you must be open and frank enough to learn or talk about this silence of meditation which I have been introducing throughout the world. I do not assume to be a teacher. We are eternal learners and yoga, as this book may help you to understand, is infinite knowledge.

Om Shanti, Shanti, Shanti

WHAT IS YOGA ALL ABOUT?

Now that you are advancing with Yoga you will have soaked up, almost incidentally, some of the many other elements of Yoga. Perhaps you are even into meditation and are slowly discovering its great joy, its marvellous resting qualities; or, your new body awareness has sparked an interest in natural nutrition. But surely you will have realized that, no matter what your original goal, you have received numerous other benefits. If it was beauty you were after you will also have received better health—suddenly the annoying bursitis, which you hadn't especially concentrated on correcting, was gone as well. Or, while you were successfully slimming, you gradually began noticing that lately you also seemed to have boundless energy. Since Yoga yokes the mind, the spirit and the body, physical health improvement also spells better mental health, greater energy, a more positive outlook on life and a relaxed and peaceful state of mind. By bending and stretching the spinal vertebrae, you not only give them a rejuvenating massage, you also increase the circulation to the spinal cord which in turn favourably influences the central nervous system. The ancient Yogis believed that our psychological and spiritual well being is closely connected with the spine. By performing the inverted postures, which truly seem to be the panacea for most ills, you receive benefit after benefit—too numerous to mention here. You are offsetting the gravitational pull, relieving congested blood vessels in some areas, and improving circulation where it normally tends to be shut off.

Why did I write this book? To guide you gently towards greater relaxation, towards awakening your dormant powers through exercise and Yoga nutrition, to lead you a little further on the royal path of self-awareness. If you have done little or no Yoga before, but find that these exercises are not too difficult, if you can touch your fingers to the floor immediately or perform a beautiful lotus on your first try—don't feel smug, you may simply have long arms or an inherently wide scope in your hip socket. The true test of flexibility is to touch your head to your knees eventually. That comes with slow but persistent efforts to release tension through stretching, with lubricating "rusty" joints, with oxygenating tired blood. Anyone of any age can start Yoga and have spectacular results. One does not "tackle" Yoga, one embraces it. The art and science of it was devised 5000 years ago to realize each individual's full potential. Yoga is highly individual—personally progressive—it is never competitive. The man who came to one of my classes, saw me sit in the Lotus position and took an attitude of "if she can do it, so can I" had not grasped the true Yoga spirit. And he suffered for his senseless competition. For, as he quickly forced his second leg onto the first thigh, he let out an enraged yell and shortly after was lifted up by the ambulance attendants, still locked in his Lotus position, and ignominiously carried away.

The essence of physical Yoga practice, then, is not to strain, but instead to bring out the natural beauty, the natural strength of your body slowly. With Yoga there is grace, balance, poise. One moves into the poses gently, holds them for as long as comfort permits, releases the position slowly and then relaxes for as long as is necessary, breathing abdominally. The advanced student simply holds a position longer—and then has to do it only once. What energy is thus released from its prison of tense muscles and joints, once they are warmed up and stretched! Yoga is a "miracle-drug" for our "instant", "super", "now" society. Instead of popping a pill to "maybe" relieve a headache, a pain in the neck or indigestion in an hour, doctor yourself up for truly instant relief with Yoga. I mean just that. Have you tried it at all? Have you relaxed into a Forward Bend for your pounding head, performed a Chest Expander for tight, tense shoulders, or the Knees-To-The-Chest for stomach gas? Have you practised Deep Breathing immediately on the onset of the trouble instead of sobbing with misery? Such therapy is what Yoga must be used for as well, besides its other functions. "Pop" Yoga, not pills, for instant relief!

My personal experience with Yoga is closely connected with the energizing and, paradoxically, the calming properties of Yoga breathing. People are incredulous, hearing that I was once twenty pounds overweight, horribly depressed and quite the hypochondriac. With the help of the Alternate Nostril Breath I was able to rid myself of the tired Housewife syndrome, with the aid of Yoga postures such as the Shoulderstand I reduced the excess weight, with the Triangle and similar postures I trimmed and firmed all over.

Of the three main areas of Hatha Yoga—body-cleansing practices, physical exercises and breathing—the latter is of the greatest importance, because air is our most important food for both body and mind. In the Sanskrit language of the ancient Yogis, breath control is called PRANAYAMA. Prana means "breath" or, more accurately, "life-force", and ayama means "pause" or "control". The Yogis believe in an invisible cosmic force around us, the mysterious essence which gives us life, a kind of universal energy. Without prana you are dead; the more you have of it, the more alive and energetic you are. By mastering proper breathing techniques, you increase your "living potential". You can become more alert and aware—master of yourself. With the help of different kinds of breathing exercises you can actually decrease appetite, soothe tired feet, or regain the spring of youth; you can "take a tranquilizer" of several breaths; you may make yourself wide-awake and alert or overcome insomnia; oxygenating the bloodstream purifies it, aids the digestion, slows down the heartbeat. I remember well the thin young woman of thirty-three who was sent to the resort hotel in Harrison Hot Springs by her doctor as a last-ditch effort to get her to relax. She was near a state of collapse because of severe insomnia and nothing seemed to help. I was teaching there at the time and carefully instructed her in the Alternate Nostril Breath. She was skeptical but so desperate that she earnestly followed instructions at bedtime. That night for the first time in months she slept! From one day to the next she bloomed—her insomnia was gone and its psychological pressure was off.

The benefits of Yoga are very much to the mind as well as to the body. How can the two possibly be separated? Yoga seeks to unite them with the spirit. All three will then work together towards the common goal of samadhi: the ultimate bliss consciousness, a sort of super-joy, peace of mind, self-realization or whatever you wish to call it. I enjoyed the answer of my beloved guru Swami Shyam Acharya when he was asked: "But what is the kind of Yoga-meditation you are teaching if it is not 'Transcendental Meditation'?" With a mischievous twinkle in his wise eyes he replied "Super Transcendental Meditation." All meditation is transcendental. The techniques are as numerous and as various as the Yoga postures. One of the most common is the use of a "mantra". This is a mystical syllable or one of the holy names of God used to set up good vibrations and as a tool to keep the restless mind from wandering. Such a word is soundlessly chanted over and over in the meditator's mind. However, no unnecessary energy is expended in pushing away persistent thoughts. One simply watches them drift past and then resumes the chanting of the mantra. Half an hour of such practice has wonderful resting properties—similar to several hours' sleep. The objective is to awaken Kundalini power which is a form of energy coiled in the base of the spine. As the Kundalini rises in the spine it next moves through six centres of spiritual energy and after years of persistent efforts with the help of a competent teacher, it finally reaches the highest centre in the brain. Cosmic Consciousness, eternal love, and absolute joy have then been achieved.

It remains now to speak of a more neglected but highly pertinent aspect of Yoga: nutrition. Most true Yogis are vegetarian. This ties in with their non-violent attitude to all life. To the Yogi meat products are a secondary protein source. He maintains that the biggest and longest living animals, such as the elephant, are vegetarian. He is very careful to get lots of protein in the form of soya beans, nuts and dairy products—a matter which many a "new" vegetarian neglects. If you stop eating meat, you must substitute with another protein source! Generally speaking a Yoga diet is simply a totally natural attitude towards permanent good health and towards the upkeep of the perfect weight for YOU. Nutrition is discussed in eye-opening detail in a later chapter and excellent nutrition books are available in most health food stores. You cannot be interested only in a losing diet, however. Once the weight is off, your whole attitude to food, to calories and towards the refrigerator must change as well, or you will simply commit yourself to a horrible not-so-merry-go-round of "off", "on", "off", "on". Since I became nutrition-conscious through Yoga, I constantly amaze myself with what I *don't* want to eat anymore. Chocolate (Hershey and German) was a MUST before. Life could not be imagined without it. Now, I do not deny it to myself entirely but the times of indulgence are few and far between, and one or two small pieces satisfy the craving that only a whole bar or two could fulfill before. My favourite snack from morning to night is mild Danish Tilsit cheese, with grapes if possible. By looking at most Woman's Magazines we can see how weight conscious our society is: the perfect, NEW diet is constantly advertised. However, deep down we know that there is no cure-all, no easy-way-out without common sense. "FASTING" is a dirty word to many people—I remember recoiling with fright from the very thought. Now I know from conversations with doctors, from my reading and personal experience with fasting that its effects are nothing short of miraculous. Fasting has a fantastic body-cleansing effect, it has marvellous resting qualities for the body, it rids the body of toxins, clears the mind as well as the skin, deflates a paunch like a burst balloon and despite its bad reputation is not at all harmful for most people. Look at any sick animal. It crawls into a hole and refuses to eat. Look at the great teacher and reformer Gandhi—fasting was a way of life for him, and he was so full of energy that he rarely slept. Closer to home, look at the Doukhobour women who fast for weeks on end, none the worse for it. Listen to Dick Gregory on the talk shows. He fasts for months yet feels wonderful. If you are weak-willed you can start with a compromise fast: water the first day, fruit juice the second, fruit the third. A slight headache at first is the only discomfort. Fasting is an excellent way to start a diet, but what happens next? To start with a breakfast high in protein is essential. A raw vegetable-salad with two tablespoons, of unsaturated salad oil (yes, oil can help you lose pounds—see Fats in Nutrition chapter) with protein for lunch, and a very light supper of milk, cheese and fruit. And do learn the difference between calories: a 350 calorie avacado is not nearly so fattening as a piece of banana cream pie which has the same number of calories, largely because the avocado has so many useful nutrients and the pie has only a few.

Nutrition, meditation, breath-control, relaxation and beauty are only a few of Yoga's aspects. Another is a feeling of good will towards one's fellow man. No one book did more towards making me a better Christian than Paramahansa Yogananda's "AUTOBIOGRAPHY OF A YOGI". After reading it I understood for the first time the significance of the story of Adam and Eve. Yoga seems to be a sort of gospel, something that really fulfills what it promises, and one wants to spread the good word. Anyone could, after proper study, be a Yoga teacher, just as anyone can invent a new Yoga pose for his own particular need, as long as the Yoga principle of slow movement and a holding position is adhered to. Marcia Moore, whose book started me on Yoga, can be credited with a new and excellent posture which she discovered through a misprint of an original pose. Yoga does not only make you flexible, it is adaptable in itself. Intelligence is the ability to adapt yourself to new situations on the basis of your experience. Be intelligent—experience Yoga up all its many steps to higher awareness of self.

BASICS OF HATHA YOGA

No matter what your age, Yoga can help you realize your secret bodily desire, be it energy, health, beauty, youthfulness or graceful bearing—if you practise regularly and sensibly. There is no doubt that Yoga can work miracles.But the instrument through which wonders are worked is you. Without your discipline, your faith in what you are doing and your persistence in doing it, there can be no results. There is a right and a wrong way of practising Yoga and often a little variation will make all the difference. Try to come to the practice of Yoga without preconceived notions of how to do the exercise. Read or listen to instructions fully and to the end. Too often people will listen half-way, think they know what is going to be said next, and go ahead and do their own incomplete and/or incorrect effort.

Practise regularly, even if you have time for only a few exercises on some days. Then, do only those that you know do *you* the most good. If you suffer from tension, do the Chest Expander; if your tummy is flabby, concentrate on the Pump, and so on. But make Yoga as much of your daily routine as eating and sleeping. The change in your health and outlook on life will make it worthwhile a hundred times over.

Never hurry. Go into the postures *slowly,* taking 10-15 seconds to get from the beginning to the holding position. This gives bonus benefits and makes each exercise more effective. It also helps to cut down on the number of times an exercise has to be done.

Hold each position once you have gone as far into it as comfort permits. Muscles must receive sustained strain in order to stay in condition. As a beginner, hold each posture at its extremity for 5 seconds. Increase this time by 5 seconds a week as you improve. Through the holding position you are doing an exercise over and over as it were, and therefore an excercise need be done only three times, instead of twenty.

Come out of an exercise as slowly as you went into it. You lose at least a third of the value if you permit yourself to collapse, and you might even risk injury.

Never force a position, never jerk or bounce in order to "go further". Go as far as you can, then hold it there. Pain is a danger-signal devised by the body to stop immediately or risk injury. If, as in calisthenics, you are moving so fast that your momentum does not permit you to stop short, you can easily move past the danger-signal and get hurt. This is what happens when you experience muscular soreness or muscle-strain.

Never compare yourself to anyone else. Yoga emphasizes "Personal Progress." By performing the exercise regularly you are bound to do better today than you did yesterday. In going to the limit of your capability you receive the same benefits as your teacher who can stretch much further but who is also more flexible. In Yoga there is visible progress. You will find that after a time you can get into poses you would never have dreamed possible.

Concentrate intensely with each exercise you perform. It will follow naturally that you then do the exercise well. This is especially necessary in balancing exercises. Moving your head rapidly, or speaking or laughing embarrassedly when you do lose your balance will retard your progress and efficiency. Simply carry on where you left off without a feeling of disgust or embarrassment at yourself. Then your concentration will remain unbroken and you can achieve much. Visualizing encourages concentration which in turn promotes quality of action. For instance, pretend to be a fierce lion in the Lion or a pussy-cat just up from her nap in the Cat Stretch. It will make exercising more fun for you too.

Rest between exercises. The beauty of Yoga lies in its gentleness. You need never experience draining fatigue or painful, sore muscles. Catch your breath, let the muscles rebound from a delightful stretch and permit the body to assimilate what it has learned.

Breathe normally during the holding position of an exercise. There is a tendency for most people to hold their breath while they desperately and tensely hold on. This is absolutely wrong. Yoga stresses relaxation, even while exercising. If at all possible, you should go as far into a pose as comfort permits, then relax there and breathe normally. As a student advances in proficiency there is a prescribed way of breathing with each exercise.

Always keep your body relaxed even at the apex of a position, except for those parts which are directly involved in the pose. For example, in the Cobra concentrate on the back and keep the buttocks and thighs relaxed. The effort you are making should never be mirrored in a distorted face.

The best time to exercise is either first thing in the morning or last thing at night. It depends on your particular need. In the morning the body is still stiff, but the exercises will help you to work better all day. In the evening the exercising comes more easily and refreshes and relaxes you for a good sleep.

A private, airy place where you can expect little interruption is best. For, the more you concentrate, the better you will do each exercise. A rug or a blanket folded in four will give you good protection from the hard floor without being too soft for efficient performance.

It is wise not to eat a heavy meal for at least 2 hours before exercising strenuously. It is permissible to take a light meal or a little liquid.

Always empty the bladder and move the bowels before the practice of Yoga. The Yoga postures are done more easily after a bath, especially if you are a tense or arthritic person. You will find that constipation is no longer a problem with regular practice, but since the upside-down poses promote elimination, it is advisable to start your program with these.

Ladies, you may exercise during menstruation if you wish—on a lighter scale than normal, however. Only practise the inverted postures such as the Shoulderstand, if no pains or changes in the amount of flow result. It is quite safe to practise Yoga during pregnancy for the first three months, or longer, but you should always check with your doctor first. There are special exercises to make the muscles of the back strong and elastic, to strengthen the floor of the pelvis, and to master deep breathing techniques as aids to labour.

People with High Blood Pressure, Dizziness or Detached Retina should always check with their doctor. They should not at first do any of the inverted postures such as the ShoulderStand, but any of the forward bending poses are beneficial. To experience a certain amount of dizziness in the beginning is quite normal, since the head usually gets little circulation. In the inverted postures there is a sudden onrush of blood dilating the blood vessels, and a slight headache or dizziness may result.

Even after a knee-shaking Yoga work-out, you will not suffer from muscular soreness if you follow the sensible rules laid out here. For maximum benefit with a minimum effort, please consider all these points every time you practise Yoga.

YOGA EXERCISES

(ASANAS)

ABDOMINAL LIFT (UDDIYANA BANDHA)

I. *Benefits:*

The Abdominal Lift . . .
- strengthens and firms the *abdominal muscles.*
- reduces the *waistline.*
- promotes *regularity* and relieves *constipation* by stimulating the peristaltic action of the colon.
- tones and massages most *abdominal organs* and *glands.*
- improves circulation to the abdominal area which aids the *digestion* and *metabolism.*

II. *Technique:*

1. Stand straight, the legs about a foot apart.
2. Bend forward placing your hands just above the knees and shifting your weight onto them. (The hands may be placed wherever it is most comfortable for you.)
3. Inhale and then EXHALE FULLY and do not breathe again throughout the exercise. It is of the greatest importance that no breath should be left in the body.
4. Relax the abdomen and pull it inward and then upward as though to have the navel touch the spine. This creates a deep hollow. (Figure 1)
5. Hold the inward pull for as long as you can and then bang the abdomen out in a sudden motion.
6. Relax and inhale.
7. Repeat steps one to six at least three times.
8. When you have mastered the idea of pulling the abdomen in on an *exhalation,* with not a vestige of breath left in the body, go on with step 9—but only then.
9. After pulling the relaxed abdomen in and up, hold the inward pull for one second and then bang the abdomen suddenly.
10. Immediately pull the abdomen in again, remembering to also give the upward pull which should be so strong that it tightens the muscles of the neck.
11. Bang the abdomen out again after one second, etc.
12. Repeat this in and out motion for a total of 3-10 times on the one exhalation.
13. Relax, gasping for air. If you find that you are exhaling as you straighten out, you will have done the exercise wrong.
14. Perform a set of 3-5 contractions each three times and if you are really concerned about constipation or slack muscles, then do this three times a day.

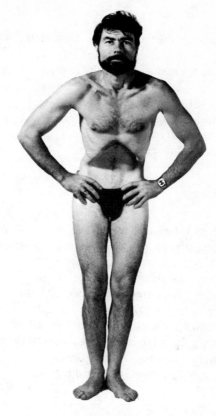

(Figure 1)

III. *Dos and Don'ts:*

DO make sure that your lungs are completely empty before pulling the abdomen in. This will take a little practice and you may find that you tend to breathe in with each inward pull. The 3-5 contractions are all performed on one breath.

DO have your abdomen relaxed to permit a proper hollowing.

DO work up your contractions to 10 on one exhalation as you advance, but do it gradually at one extra contraction a week.

DO NOT get discouraged if your abdomen is fat and doesn't seem to hollow at all. That emaciated look will just take a little longer to achieve, but it will happen.

DO practice this pose in front of a mirror.

VARIATION: NAULI

I. *Benefits:*

- most effectively corrects digestive problems such as *constipation* and *indigestion.*
- encourages normal action of the *liver.*
- massages the *kidneys, spleen* and *pancreas.*
- relieves painful *periods.*
- strengthens *abdominal muscles.*
- rids the *intestinal tract* of toxins.
- helps with *sexual debility.*

II. *Technique:*

1. Perform steps 1-4 as above as in Abdominal Lift.
2. Now concentrate on pushing the recti muscles in the middle of the abdomen forward, while keeping the rest of the abdomen hollowed.
3. Hold the position; relax and inhale. (Figure 2)
4. When you have mastered this rather difficult task, go on to:
5. Performing steps 1-4 as in Abdominal Lift.
6. Now *concentrate* on pushing out the left rectus muscles (not to be confused with the rectum, or lowest part of the intestines) alone.
7. Do the same on the right side. (Figure 3)
8. Hold each position, then relax and inhale.
9. When this deliberate isolation is well-established, try to perform a churning pose from left to right or vice versa, through several rounds.

III. *Dos and Don'ts:*

DON'T get discouraged if you do not succeed in your efforts at first—this is a most difficult pose to perform.

DO "bear forward" similar to the "bearing down" of child-birth, or a difficult bowel movement.

DO relax first and only then try again if you "simply can't get it right".

DO NOT practice Nauli lightly—it is only for the advanced students and should not be practiced by children, people over 40, or anyone with abdominal diseases or high blood pressure.

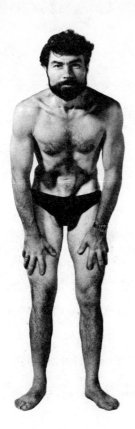

(Figure 2)

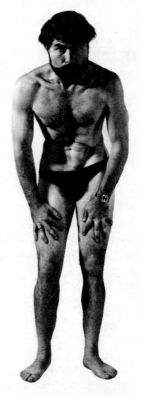

Duncan McDougall Age 42

(Figure 3)

THE ANKLE TO FOREHEAD STRETCH (EKA PADA SIRSASANA)

I. *Benefits:*

The Ankle to Forehead Stretch. . .
- is beneficial to the *hip joints.*
- stretches and firms the *thighs* and *hip muscles.*
- relieves *sciatica.*
- strengthens the *arms.*
- massages the *abdominal organs* and improves *digestion.*
- raises a *"slipped hip".*

II. *Technique:*

1. Sit, legs outstretched.
2. Bend the right leg bringing the foot close to the body, letting the knee fall to the side.
3. From underneath grasp the right foot around the ankle with the right hand.
4. Get a good grasp around the ball of the foot with the left hand. (Figure 4)
5. EXHALE, raise the foot as high as you can or on a level with the face.
6. Bend the head forward and pull the ankle to the forehead or as close as possible. (Figure 5)
7. Hold the pose for 5-30 seconds, breathing normally. EXHALE, relax.
8. Repeat on the other side.

Variation 1: (very advanced)

1. Steps 1 and 2 as above.
3. Grasp the right ankle with both hands, pulling the foot up.
4. EXHALE, bend slightly forward and slowly bring the right foot up and back, lifting it over the head onto the back of the neck. (Figure 6)
5. Straighten the head and neck and bring the palms together in front of the chest.
6. Hold 5-30 seconds, breathing normally.
7. Repeat on the other side.

III. *Dos and Don'ts:*

DO bend your trunk forward at first to get the ankle and the forehead together. Straighten the trunk as you improve.

DO keep the other leg straight.

DO NOT attempt the variation until you are proficient in the Ankle to Forehead Stretch.

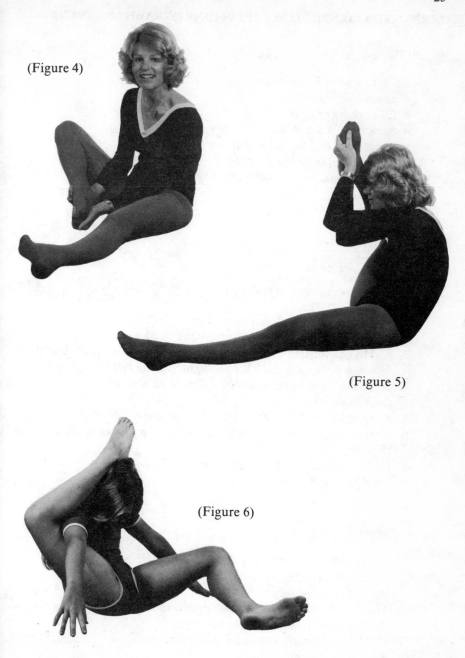

(Figure 4)

(Figure 5)

(Figure 6)

This exercise gives a delightful stretching sensation to the whole hip region and has a slimming effect as well.

*ARM AND LEG STRETCH VARIATIONS (VIRABHADRASANA)

I. *Benefits:*

Arm & Leg Stretch Variations . . .
- make *legs* shapely.
- fill in *skinny thighs.*
- *reduce fat* in the *hips.*
- facilitate breathing for *asthma* sufferers.
- reduce *tension* and stiffness of the *neck, shoulders* and *back.*
- are beneficial to the *ankles* and *knees.*
- relieve *leg cramps.*
- tone the *abdominal organs.*

II. *Technique:*

Variation 1:

1. Stand, the feet four feet apart.
2. INHALE, joining the palms above the head.
3. EXHALE, turning the body towards the right, and swivelling the right foot to a 90° angle, the left foot slightly to the right. (Figure 7)
4. Bend the right knee, until the thigh is parallel to the floor forming a right angle with the shin.
5. Keep the left leg straight, tightening the knee.
6. Stretch the arms and then the spine up, looking at the hands. (Figure 8)
7. Hold 5-30 seconds, breathing normally.
8. EXHALE and relax. Repeat on the other side.

Variation 2:

1. Stand, the feet four feet apart.
2. INHALE, raise the arms parallel to the floor, palms down.
3. Repeat steps 3-5 as above.
6. Turn the head to the right and stretch the hands away from you. Keep the body in a straight line. (Figure 9)
7. Hold 5-30 seconds, breathing normally.
8. Repeat on the other side.

*Basic exercise described in ABC of Yoga

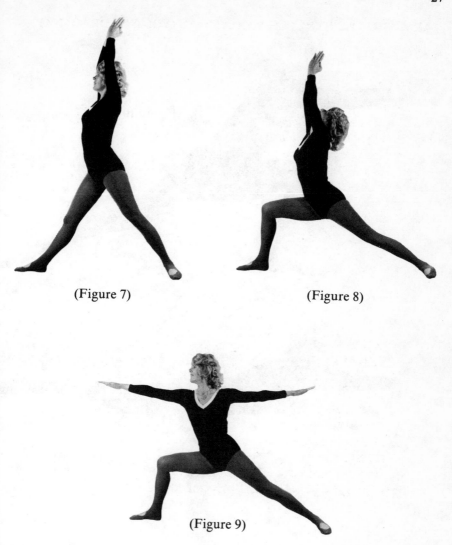

(Figure 7)   (Figure 8)

(Figure 9)

III. *Dos and Don'ts:*

DO keep the knee of the stretched-out leg tight.
DO get a good opposite stretch between the legs and the hands, as though
   you were being pulled apart.

The Standing poses should be mastered by all beginners, as they strengthen
and prepare for more advanced forward bending poses. Until strength is built
up, however, it suffices to do the simple Triangle Poses. All these have a
reducing effect.

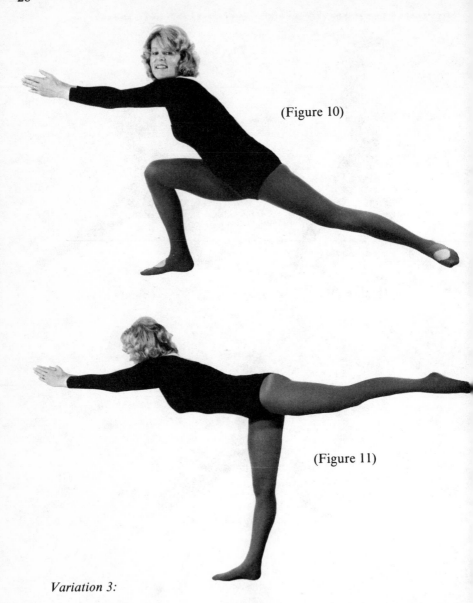

(Figure 10)

(Figure 11)

Variation 3:

1. Repeat steps 1-5 as in Variation 1.
6. EXHALE, bend forward and rest the chest on the knee. Breathe two
   normal breaths. (Figure 10)
7. EXHALE, and raise the *left* leg parallel to the floor.
8. At the same time, straighten the right knee, tilting the body forward.
9. Hold 5-20 seconds, breathing normally. (Figure 11)
10. Stretch the hands and the feet away from each other.
11. EXHALE, relax and repeat on the other side.

*BOW VARIATIONS (PADANGUSTHA DHANURASANA)

I. *Benefits:*

Bow Variations . . .
- strengthen and limber up the *lumbar* and *sacroiliac* regions of the spine.
- tone and tighten the muscles of the *abdomen, arms* and *legs.*
- reduce weight in *hips* and *buttocks.*
- improve *posture.*
- develop and firm the *muscles* of the *chest* and *bustline.*
- relieve pain from a *slipped disc.*
- aid *digestion.*

II. *Technique:*

Variation 1: Bow-To-The-Side.
1. Lie face down on the floor, hands by your side.
2. Bend your knees and bring them close to the buttocks.
3. Grab your legs at the ankles, one at a time.
4. EXHALE, lift your knees off the floor by pulling the ankles *away* from the hands.
5. Lift your head and chest at the same time balancing on the abdomen. Take 2 normal breaths.
6. EXHALE and roll over to the right side, keeping a good tight grip on the ankles. (Figure 12)
7. Hold 5-15 seconds breathing normally.
8. INHALE and come back to the Bow.
9. EXHALE and relax. Repeat on the other side.
10. Roll to both sides without rest if you are more advanced.

(Figure 12)

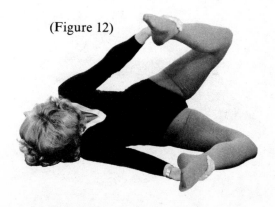

Variation 2: Cobra-Bow.

1. Lie face down on the floor, hands under the shoulders, palms down.
2. Bend the right knee, and grasp the ankle with the right hand.
3. EXHALE and lift the right knee off the floor by pulling away from the hand. (Figure 13)
4. Now INHALE and push down on the left hand, letting the head and trunk bend slowly back as in the Cobra. The arm slides slightly forward.
5. Hold, breathing normally for 5-10 seconds. (Figure 14)
6. EXHALE and slowly relax.
7. Repeat on the other side.

Variation 3: Crossed Bow

1. Lie face down on the floor, hands by your side.
2. Bend your knees, crossing the ankles and bring the heels close to the buttocks.
3. Grasp the crossed feet closest to the reach, one at a time.
4. EXHALE. Lift your knees off the floor by pulling the ankles *away* from the hands. Hold on tightly all the while.
5. Lift your head and chest at the same time. (Figure 15)
6. Hold the position 5-15 seconds, increasing to 30 seconds at 5 seconds a week. Breathe normally.
7. EXHALING, slowly relax and rest for awhile.
8. Repeat twice more.

Variation 4:
Rock gently in a normal Bow pose.

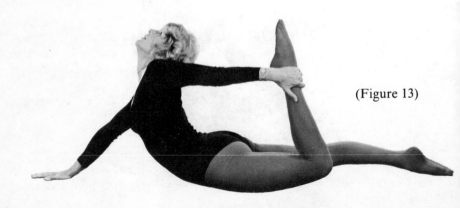

(Figure 13)

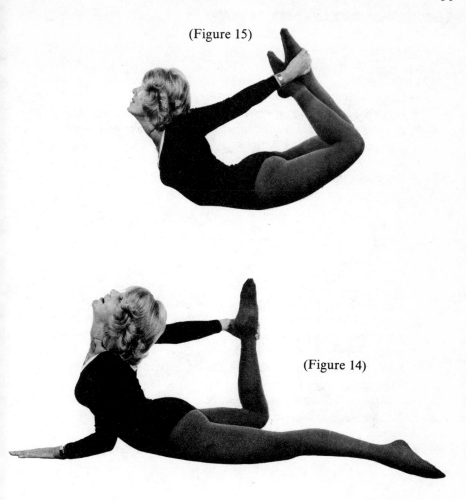

(Figure 15)

(Figure 14)

III. *Dos and Don'ts:*

DO pull the ankles "up and away" rather than down to master the trick of getting the knees off the floor.

DO remember to breathe normally and relax as much as possible while holding the pose.

DO NOT collapse in a heap. You will make the exercise more effective by slowly relaxing.

The Bow is a particularly useful asana because it combines the benefits of both the Cobra and the Locust. It gives back to the spine the elasticity that is so often lost with tension and age.

THE BRIDGE (UTTANA MAYURASANA)

I. *Benefits:*

The Bridge . . .
- limbers up the *spine* and makes it flexible.
- tones the *central nervous system.*
- relieves *neck strain* after such exercises as the Shoulderstand.
- tightens and firms the *buttocks.*
- strengthens the *wrists.*
- tightens and reduces *midriff* fat.

II. *Technique:*

1. Perform a Shoulderstand.
2. With the hands around the waist, thumbs to the front, bring the left leg over the head, parallel to the floor, as though to do a Plough.
3. Slowly lower the right leg to the floor in front, with the knee slightly bent, toes pointing down. The left leg follows slowly, acting as a balancing agent. (Figure 16)
4. Stretch the legs out as much as possible, knees together, heels touching the floor. (Figure 17)
5. Shift your weight towards the neck.
6. Hold 15-30 seconds, eventually increasing to a minute at the rate of 5 seconds a week. Breathe normally.
7. Relax, repeat with the other leg.

Variation: Drawbridge

1. Repeat steps 1-5 as above.
6. Bend the knees again and rest your weight on the toes.
7. Lift the left leg as high as possible over the head.
8. Now attempt to lift the right leg off the floor and return to the Shoulderstand. (Figure 18)

The Bridge and the Drawbridge, in particular, are asanas of almost gymnastic calibre. Once mastered, they increase flexibility and strength and give one such a pleasant feeling of accomplishment that it is worthwhile to practise them for that reason alone.

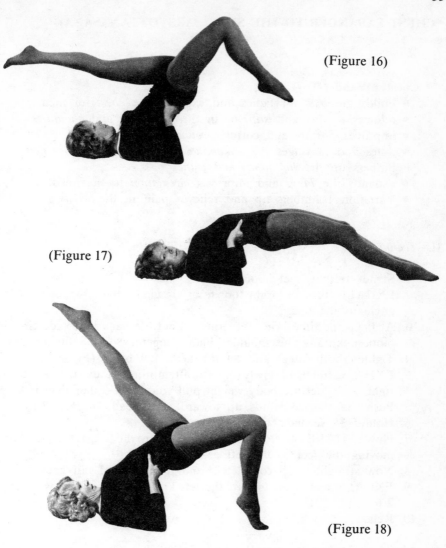

(Figure 16)

(Figure 17)

(Figure 18)

III. *Dos and Don'ts:*

DO concentrate fiercely, since this asana is largely a balancing one.
DO stretch your legs out for those extra benefits.
DO keep a tight grip on the waist throughout.
DO NOT use jerky motions, but at the beginning a slight push with the right
    foot is permitted to get you out of the Drawbridge.
DO NOT put all your weight on the wrists and elbows, but shift it towards
    the neck.

*CHEST EXPANDER-TO-THE-SIDE (PARSVOTTANASANA)

I. *Benefits:*

Chest Expander-To-The-Side . . .
- builds the *bust* for ladies and expands the *chest* for men.
- relieves *tension* and *stiffness* in the *legs, hips* and *shoulders.*
- improves *posture* and corrects *round shoulders*
- tones and massages the *abdominal organs* and aids *digestion.*
- limbers up the *hip joints* and *spine.*
- expands the *lungs* and improves *circulation* to the head.
- Variation 1 limbers up and relieves pain in the *wrists.*

II. *Technique:*
Variation 1:
1. Stand straight, feet about 3 feet apart.
2. EXHALE, turn the right foot to a 90° angle, the left foot to a 75° angle to the body.
3. At the same time bring the arms behind the back in a wide circling motion, knifing the shoulder blades together. Clasp the hands.
4. Tighten both knees and let the head fall back. (Figure 19)
5. EXHALE and bend slowly forward, attempting to touch the head to the right knee. Let the body weight pull you down rather than jerking. Push the clasped hands up toward your head. (Figure 20)
6. Hold 5-15 seconds, breathing normally.
7. Now INHALE and slowly swivel the body to the left, at the same time moving the feet to the left as in step 2.
8. Now straighten up completely and let the head fall back.
9. EXHALE and bend toward the left knee, and continue as in steps 2-6.
10. Relax.

Variation 2: The Respectful Chest Expander.
1. Stand straight, INHALE deeply and arch the back.
2. Bring the palms together in the back, fingertips pointing down.
3. EXHALE and rotate the wrists up, barely keeping the fingertips touching.
4. Move the hands up the back as much as possible. (Figure 21)
5. Proceed with the rest of the Chest Expander.

*Chest Expander is described in ABC of Yoga.

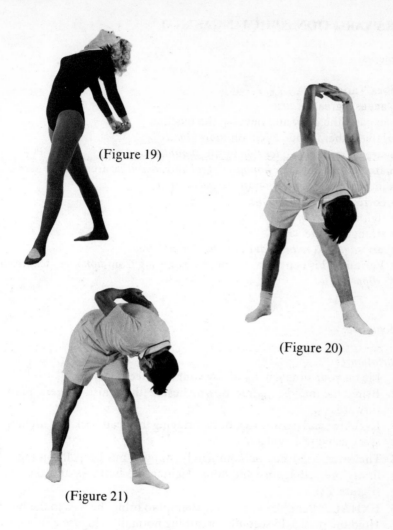

(Figure 19)

(Figure 20)

(Figure 21)

III. *Dos and Don'ts:*

DO keep the knees tightened by moving up the kneecaps.
DO steps 7 and 8 on one complete exhalation.
DO keep both knees straight.
DO NOT force the head closer to the knees than
it comfortably wants to go.
DO concentrate, however, on stretching the back.

The Chest Expander in all its variations stretches most of the body and therefore acts as a quick energizer and de-tensionizer. These variations concentrate the stretching action on the hip and leg area and whittle away the "squished-up" look of many an abdomen.

*COBRA VARIATIONS (BHUJANGASANA)

I. *Benefits:*

Cobra Variations . . .
- act as a great *vitalizer.*
- expand the *chest* and develop the bustline.
- have a therapeutic effect on *most glands.*
- stretch and relieve *tension* in the *shoulders* and *neck.*
- are beneficial to the *lumbar, dorsal* and *sacroiliac* areas of the *spine.*
- improve the *circulation* to the *pelvic* area.
- correct *urinary problems.*
- tighten the *chin* area.
- strengthen the *wrists.*
- *massage* and *reduce fat* in the *abdominal area.*
- Variation 2 is beneficial for people suffering from *lumbago, sciatica* and *slipped disc.*

II. *Technique:*

Variation 1:
1. Lie on your stomach, hands by your side, feet together.
2. Bring the hands, palms down, beside the waist, fingers pointing forward.
3. INHALE and perform a Cobra, bringing the head back and arching the spine as far as it will go.
4. The arms need not be completely straight but keep the pubic area firmly pressed against the floor. Tighten the buttocks and the thighs. (Figure 22)
5. EXHALE. Bend the knees and attempt to bring the toes to the head.
6. Hold the pose 5-15 seconds, breathing normally. (Figure 23)
7. Slowly relax, EXHALING. Repeat twice more.

III. *Dos and Don'ts:*

DO think of the spine as a heavy chain and raise this chain slowly, link by link.
DO bring the head up first and let it come down last.
DO give a good stretch to the legs and the body in this position.
DO tighten and lock the elbows and knees whenever specified.
DO NOT force any position that does not come easily.

*Cobra is described in ABC of Yoga

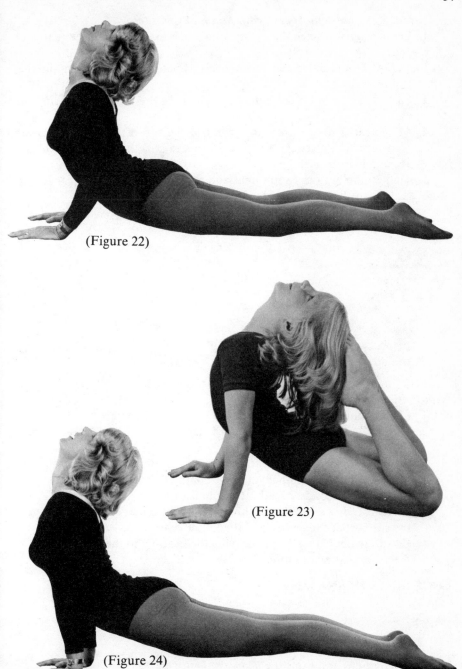

(Figure 22)

(Figure 23)

(Figure 24)

The Cobra is a classic asana and as such brings a multitude of benefits. Combined with positive thinking and an enjoyment of the movement of your own body—these benefits will be manifold.

Variation 2: Cobra-on-Toes (Urdva Mukha Svanasana)

1. Lie on your stomach, hands by your waist, palms down, feet one foot apart.
2. INHALE and raise the head, neck, shoulders and back as in the Cobra.
3. Push down hard on the hands straightening the arms and locking the elbows.
4. At the same time shift your weight to the top of the toes which are pointing straight back. Keep the legs straight, the knees locked and about 3 inches off the floor.
5. Tighten the buttocks and thighs and stretch the head back. (Figure 24)
6. Hold from 10-30 seconds breathing normally.
7. Exhale, lower the trunk and relax. Repeat twice more.

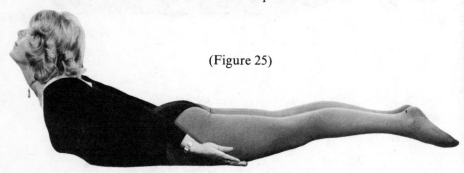

(Figure 25)

Variation 3: Cobra Without Hands

1. Lie on your stomach hands by your side, palms up.
2. INHALE, and slowly raise the head, neck and shoulders and as much of the back as your strength permits.
3. When you can go no further, bring the hands palm down beside the waist and let them help you to do a complete Cobra. (Figure 25)
4. Hold 10-30 seconds, breathing normally.
5. EXHALE, lower the trunk slowly until you think you no longer need the support of the hands, and then remove them.
6. Continue the Cobra slowly, leaving the head up to the very last.
7. Relax, repeat twice more.

COCK (KUKKUTANASANA)

I. *Benefits:*

The Cock. . .
- strengthens and firms the *abdominal muscles.*
- strengthens the *wrists.*
- promotes *balance* and therefore *poise.*
- exercises the *knees.*
- is beneficial to the *urinary system.*

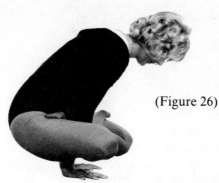

(Figure 26)

The Cock, once the Lotus position is mastered, is a deceptively easy position and fun to show off.

II. *Technique:*

1. Sit, legs outstretched.
2. Bring the right foot to the left thigh.
3. Bend the left knee, grasp the foot with both hands and lift it gently onto the right thigh.
4. Move the right foot slightly forward from under the left leg.
5. Place your left hand in between the triangular space created by the left leg, fingers pointing forward.
6. With the right hand, lift the right foot onto the left leg, forming a full lotus.
7. Place the right hand through the triangular opening formed by the right leg. Place the hands as close together as possible.
8. EXHALE, bend slightly forward and lift the buttocks off the floor, balancing on the hands. Breathe normally. (Figure 26)
9. EXHALE, lower the body, relax. Repeat, with the legs crossed the other way.

Variation 1:
1. Perform a full lotus first.
2. Now push your pointed fingers through the triangular openings created by the legs.
3. Continue with steps 8 and 9.

III. *Dos and Don'ts:*

DO practice the Crow and Cobra if you find your wrists weak.
DO have the fingers spread slightly, for a broader balancing base.
DO have the two hands as close together as possible.
DO NOT force the knees if they do not bend readily.

COW HEAD POSE (GOMUKKHASANA)

I. *Benefits:*

The Cow Head Pose. . .
- removes *leg cramps.*
- eases the pain of *bursitis.*
- improves *posture* and *rounded shoulders.*
- firms and strengthens the *upper arms.*
- eases *tension* in the *shoulders.*
- oils the *shoulder joints (eases arthritis).*
- expands the *chest to ease breathing.*
- tones the *leg muscles.*
- improves *circulation* to the *head.*

II. *Technique:*

1. Kneel and sit on the heels, hands by your side on the floor. (Figure 27)
2. Shift your weight to the left and stretch the right leg to the front.
3. Now shift your weight onto the right hand and, bending the right knee, bring the right thigh over the left thigh.
4. Bend the right leg back, attempting to have the ankles meet, toes pointing back. Find your balance and rest your weight on the heels. (Figure 28)
5. Perform the Posture Clasp by bringing the left hand behind your back and up as far as it will go, palm facing outward.
6. Lift your right hand straight up and bend it at the elbow, bringing the hand to the centre of the back.
7. Try to get the two hands close enough together to interlock with the fingers, by partly inching them together. (Figure 29)
8. Hold the position 10-30 seconds, trying a gentle upward pull with the right hand, then a downward pull with the left.
9. Repeat on the other side with both the legs and the arms. Repeat twice more.

III. *Dos and Don'ts:*

DO practice the second half of the Cow Head Pose in the bath or the shower with your arms lathered up with soap, to ease sliding them up your back.

DO keep your back straight.

DO try using a kerchief to bridge the gap between your two hands and to give the upward and downward pull.

DO NOT strain beyond a point of comfort.

DO NOT get discouraged if one side is less flexible than the other, this is quite natural. Just concentrate on that side.

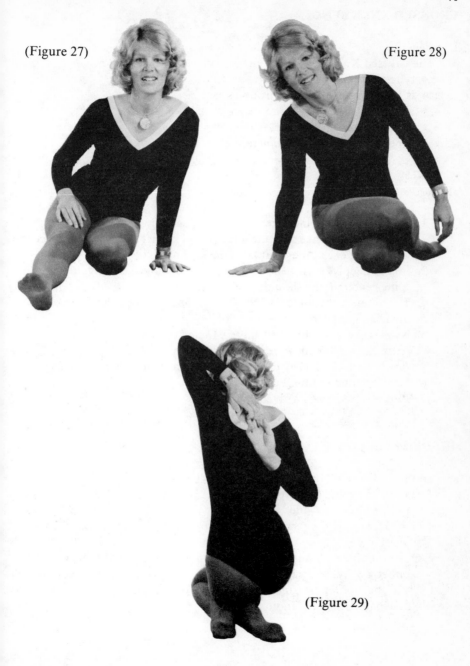

(Figure 27)

(Figure 28)

(Figure 29)

The Cow Head Pose is a quick tension reducer, especially if a lot of your time is spent hunched over a desk. It improves your posture which has a positive effect on your energy level and removes the tension from a brittle back.

CROSSED KNEE BEND

I. *Benefits:*

The Crossed Knee Bend . . .
- relieves *morning backache.*
- is excellent for *sacroiliac* troubles.
- effectively relieves gas and *indigestion.*
- is a good *breathing exercise* in its own right.
- is perfect as an *introduction* to the *Abdominal Lift.*

II. *Technique:*

1. Stand, with the spine erect.
2. Cross the right knee over the left one and keep it slightly bent. Place the toes beside each other, but keep the heel up.
3. Inhale deeply, then bend slowly forward while exhaling, keeping the spine centered, the shoulders straight.
4. Try to touch the fingers to the floor or as far as you can. Relax, letting the head hang loosely. (Figure 30)
5. Now make sure that you have *exhaled completely*, then deliberately *relax* the abdomen. A few seconds will pass, then the abdomen will slowly be sucked in by the vacuum you have created by exhaling.
6. Straighten up gradually and inhale.
7. Repeat three times with each leg.

III. *Dos and Don'ts:*

DO use a low stool or hassock, at first, to give you confidence.

DO keep the spine centered throughout the pose. Avoid the tendency to push a hip to the side.

DO NOT round the shoulders and bend the hips; bend from the waist only.

DO persist, if the tummy does not want to be sucked in at first. You a) are either not relaxing it, b) have not exhaled completely, or c) are not waiting the few seconds of complete relaxation it takes to have this fascinating phenomenon happen.

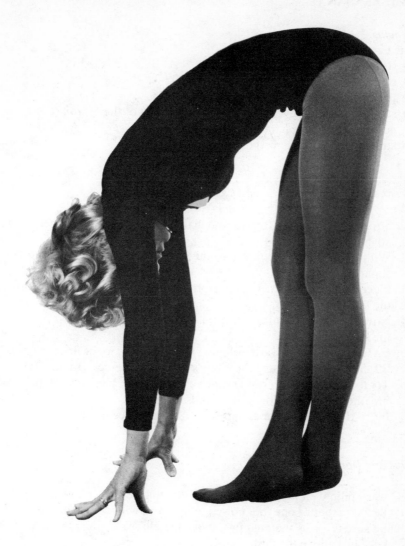

(Figure 30)

The Crossed Knee Bend, originally described as a Breathing Exercise, has been subsequently found extremely useful in relieving stomach gas. Use it NOW, when uncomfortable.

CROW (BAKASANA)

I. *Benefits:*

The Crow . . .
- strengthens and firms the *abdomen.*
- strengthens *arms* and *wrists.*
- promotes *balance* and *poise.*
- strengthens and develops the *pectoral muscles* of the *bustline.*
- acts as a *preparation* to the *Headstand.*
- strengthens the *neck* without undue pressure.

II. *Technique:*

1. Squat on the heels, feet about half a foot apart, (or together, for advanced students).
2. With the arms on the inside of the knees, rise onto the toes and bend slightly forward.
3. Place the hands on the floor in front of you, the thumbs about 6″ apart, the fingers spread slightly.
4. Now press the area of the arms just above the elbow against the side of the knee.
5. EXHALE, bend forward, bringing the face closer to the floor and gently lift the toes off, pressing the elbows against the knees. (Figure 31)
6. Try to straighten the arms as much as possible and balance on the hands breathing normally for 5-20 seconds.
7. EXHALE, lower the toes and relax. Repeat twice more.

III. *Dos and Don'ts:*

DO use a pillow on the floor in front of you to give you confidence.
DO keep the toes of one foot poised to help you with your balance.
DO be sure to press the area just above the elbows against the side of the knee just above the fleshy part.

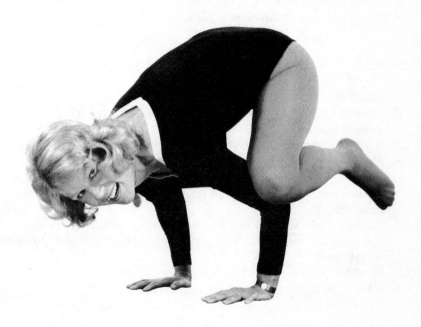

(Figure 31)

The Crow is a balancing exercise and as such requires more confidence than skill. It is easier to perform than it looks and is a good preparation for the Headstand.

DEEP LUNGE (SIRANGUSHTASANA)

I. *Benefits:*

The Deep Lunge . . .
- strengthens and firms the *thighs* and *calves.*
- strengthens *weak ankles,* excellent for skiing.
- massages and tones the *abdominal organs.*
- makes the *legs* and *ankles* shapely.
- improves the *circulation* to the *head.*
- promotes *balance* and thereby *poise.*

II. *Technique:*

1. Stand, the feet about 2½ feet apart.
2. Turn the right foot to a 90° angle to the body, the left foot pointing straight forward.
3. Bend your right knee and shift the body weight onto the right leg.
4. EXHALE, clasp your hands behind your back and bend the body forward, resting the chest on the right thigh. (Figure 32)
5. At the same time, slide the left leg back as far as possible, keeping the knee straight.
6. Having established your balance, now slowly slide the chest off the thigh on the inside and attempt to bring he head (forehead) to the floor.
7. Hold for 10-30 seconds, breathing normally. (Figure 33)
8. EXHALE, straighten up slowly and relax.
9. Repeat on the other side. Repeat on both sides twice more.

III. *Dos and Don'ts:*

DO keep the left foot pointed forward to give you a broader base of balance.

DO use the hands as support at the beginning.

DO use your body weight to help you bring the head closer to the floor, rather than jerking or forcing.

DO NOT bend your left knee.

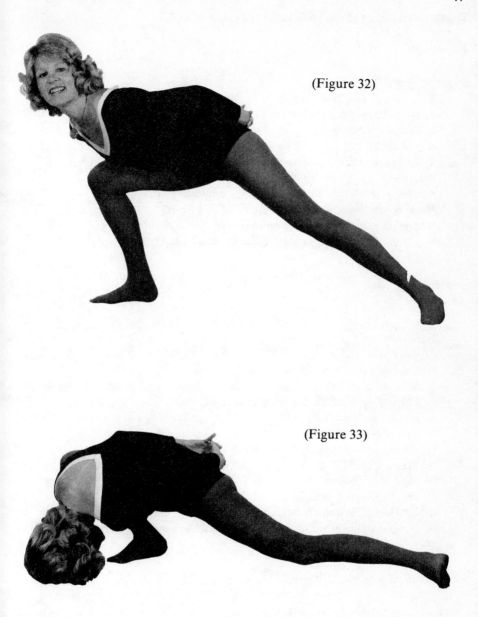

(Figure 32)

(Figure 33)

The Deep Lunge combines many benefits for the whole leg and is particularly recommended for athletes and for ladies who want the firm look for all year round.

DOG STRETCH (ADHO MUKHA SVANASANA)

I. *Benefits:*

The Dog Stretch . . .
- acts as an *energizer.*
- is a good *preparation* for the *Headstand* (as it is *safe* for people with *High Blood Pressure*).
- makes the *legs* and *ankles* shapely.
- strengthens the *abdominal muscles.*
- *slows* down the *heartbeat.*
- is recommended for *arthritis* in the *shoulder joints.*
- improves the *circulation* to the *head* and *heart.*
- relieves *stiffness* and *tension* in the *neck* and *shoulders.*
- softens *calcaneal spurs* and relieves pain in *heels.*

II. *Technique:*

1. Lie on your stomach, hands beside the shoulders, fingers pointing forward.
2. Tuck the toes under, EXHALE and push down on your hands lifting the body in a straight line as in an Army push-up.
3. When the arms are straight, bend the body at the waist and push the bottom up, shifting the weight onto the feet.
4. Move the head toward the feet and place the very top of the head on the floor. (Figure 34)
5. Keep the knees straight and push the heels toward the floor.
6. Stretch the back and keep the elbows straight, sliding the hands forward, if necessary
7. Hold the pose, breathing normally 15-60 seconds.
8. EXHALE, lower the body to the floor, and relax.
9. Repeat twice more, if you did not hold the pose for very long.

The Dog Stretch I consider one of the most important poses in Yoga. It is an invigorating pose when the energy flags, it reduces tension in almost every part of the body and has the effect of a good massage on the feet. I love it.

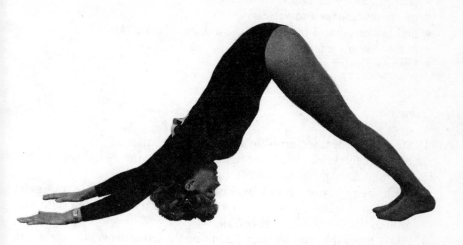

(Figure 34)

III. *Dos and Don'ts:*

   DO bend the elbows somewhat, if it is necessary in order to bring the head
      to the floor.
   DO try to do this pose in your bare feet, so that you won't slide.
   DO attempt this pose from an all-fours position at first, if your arms are too
      weak for the push-up motion.
   DO push your heels towards the floor.
   DO NOT bend the knees.
   DO remember that the Dog Stretch is a very advanced pose and as such will
      take some time to master.

EAGLE POSE (GARUDASANA)

I. *Benefits:*

The Eagle Pose . . .
- coordinates the *central nervous system.*
- promotes *balance* and *poise.*
- makes *shapely* and *strengthens* the *ankles, legs* and *thighs.*
- helps to remove *leg cramps.*
- limbers up stiff *shoulders.*

II. *Technique:*

1. Stand, feet together, arms up at the sides for balance.
2. Bend the left knee and lift the right leg, bringing the right thigh over the left thigh as high up as possible, one against the other.
3. With the right calf pressed against the side of the left knee, bring the right foot around the back of the left leg and try to curl the right toes around the left ankle. (Figure 35)
4. NOW bring the arms forward and bring the left arm over the right arm above the elbows.
5. Bend the right elbow and bring the right wrist over the left wrist, joining the hands.
6. Balance in this position for 5-15 seconds, breathing normally.
7. OR, bend your body slowly forward from the waist, with the clasped hands in front of the face, until the elbows touch the knee. (Figure 36)
8. Disengage yourself, relax. Repeat on the other side.

III. *Dos and Don'ts:*

DO practise simple balancing exercises first, if you have difficulty.
DO concentrate fiercely.
DO cross the legs up high, for an easier wrapping motion.
DO cross the arms in an opposite direction from the legs.
DO NOT attempt to bend forward until you are secure in the first part of the position.

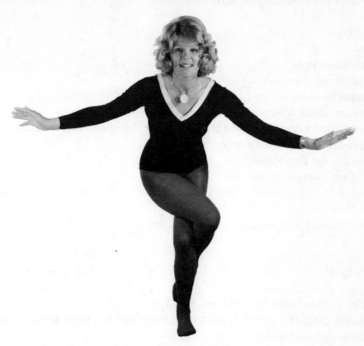

(Figure 35)

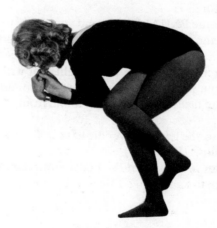

(Figure 36)

The Eagle Pose not only looks terribly impressive but has impressive results. It does take time to accomplish and needs your perseverance. One of the rewarding things in Yoga is that there are many benefits in the attempt alone.

EAR TO KNEE POSE (JANU SIRSASANA)

I. *Benefits:*

Ear to Knee Pose. . .
- acts as an *energizer.*
- tones the *spinal area* because of improved circulation.
- relieves *backache.*
- aids *digestion* and *elimination* and tones the *abdominal muscles.*
- is recommended for *kidney ailments.*
- makes the *legs shapely.*
- reduces *weight* in the *waist.*
- keeps the *pelvic area* healthy (helps to prevent enlarged prostate).
- relieves *tension.*
- Variation 1 is beneficial to the *hip joint.*

II. *Technique:*

1. Sit, legs outstretched and two feet apart.
2. Bend the left leg and bring the foot against the right thigh, letting the knee fall to the side.
3. Place the right lower arm, palm up, on the right thigh.
4. Turn your body to the left so that it is at right angles with the right leg.
5. Lift your left arm at the side and bring it slowly over your head, elbow straight. (Figure 37)
6. At the same time EXHALE and bend your body to the right, sliding the right arm to the floor on the inside of the leg and forward towards the foot.
7. Grasp the arch of the inside of the right foot with the right hand and reach over your head holding the same foot around the outside with the left hand. The face will be pointing to the front, the ear placed against the knee.
8. Hold this pose, the left arm over the left ear, for 5-20 seconds, the breath fast and shallow. (Figure 38)
9. INHALE, slowly straighten the body, and relax. Repeat on the other side.

Variation 1:
1. Sit, legs outstretched and 2 feet apart.
2. Bend the left leg and bring the foot up high on the right thigh.
3. Proceed with steps 3-8 as above. (Figure 40)

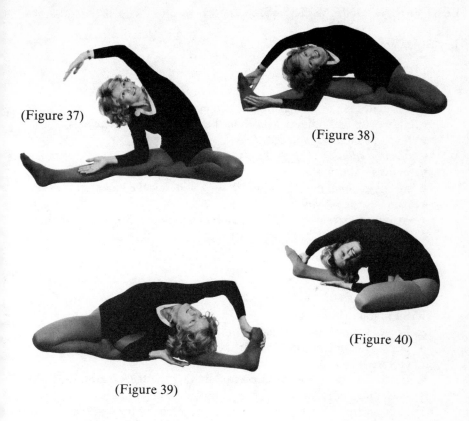

(Figure 37)

(Figure 38)

(Figure 40)

(Figure 39)

Variation 2: (Parivrtta Janu Sirsasana)
1. Follow steps 1-7.
2. Now bend and widen the elbows and twist the body completely to the left so that the back of the head rests on top of the right leg.
3. Proceed as above. (Figure 39)

III. *Dos and Don'ts:*

DO make sure that the knee is straight.
DO twist your body to the left for perfect execution of the pose and those extra benefits.
DO remember to keep the palm up throughout.

This pose, like all forward bending poses, will show you very rapid progress, with regular practice. Therefore do not get discouraged if you are nowhere near your goal at first. It should become a favourite because it has many health and beauty benefits.

FISH VARIATIONS (MATSYASANA)

I. *Benefits:*

The Fish. . .
- is beneficial for *asthma* and other *respiratory complaints.*
- stimulates the *thyroid* gland for *weight control.*
- limbers up and relieves *tension* in the *neck* and *upper back.*
- develops the *chest* and *bust line.*
- aids *digestion.*
- relieves painful *piles.*
- improves *circulation* to the *head:* for a wide-awake and alert feeling.
- exercises the *hip joints.*
- Variation 3 strengthens the *abdominal muscles,* makes the *spine* supple.

II. *Technique:*

Variation 1:
1. Sit in the Lotus position.
2. Lower yourself on the back with the aid of the elbows.
3. Slip the hands partially under the upper thigh and press down on the elbows.
4. EXHALE and push the chest up, arching the back, and pull the head back and under until you are resting on the crown of it.
5. Now grasp the legs and increase the arch of the back as much as possible. (Figure 41)
6. Lift the arms up over the head and rest them on the floor, elbows straight. (Figure 42)
7. Hold 10-60 seconds, breathing deeply.
8. INHALE, lower the body, relax. Repeat with the legs crossed the other way.

Variation 2:
1. Follow steps 1-5 as above.
6. Lift the arms over the head and cross them, holding the elbows, and attempt to lower them to the floor behind the head.
7. Repeat steps 7 and 8 as above.

The Fish is of the greatest importance for people with respiratory complaints and it should follow any pose that puts strain on the neck. The name is appropriate because one can float in this position.

Variation 3: (Uttana Padasana)
1. Lie with the legs outstretched.
2. Perform a Fish with the legs straight. (Steps 3-5) Breathe normally.
6. Now EXHALE and lift the legs up to a 45° angle off the floor.
7. Bring the arms up, palms touching, and keep them parallel to the legs.
8. Hold the pose, legs straight, for 10-30 seconds, breathing normally.
9. EXHALE, lower the body and relax. (Figure 44)

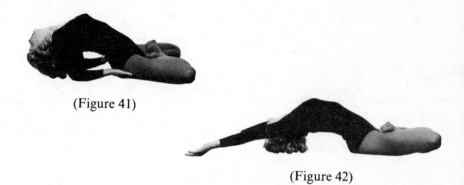

(Figure 41)

(Figure 42)

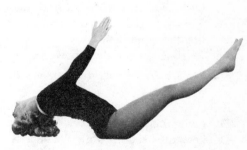

(Figure 44)

III. *Dos and Don'ts:*

DO shift your body weight to the buttocks.
DO have only the crown of the head and the buttocks touching the floor in Variation 2.
DO remember to breathe normally.
DO have positive thoughts about your weight and your health benefits while in the pose.
DO concentrate.

*FORWARD BEND STANDING VARIATIONS (UTTANASANA)

I. *Benefits:*

Forward Bend Standing Variations. . .
- improve the *posture.*
- expand the *chest* and therefore aids in the *breathing* in *respiratory ailments.*
- give an excellent *massage* to the *abdominal organs* and therefore. . .
- aid *digestion* and *elimination.*
- relieve the *pain* in *stiff* and *rheumatic knees.*
- relieve *bloating* and *flatulence.*
- are beneficial to *disc problems.*

II. *Technique:*

Variation 1: (Padangusthasana)
1. Stand, feet slightly apart.
2. EXHALE, bend forward from the waist, keeping the back concave and get a hold of the big toes between the thumb and the next 2 fingers. (Figure 45)
3. Hold for 2 breaths, then EXHALE, bend the elbows and bring the head to the knees.

Variation 2: (Pada Hastasana)
1. Stand, feet slightly apart.
2. EXHALE, bend forward from the waist, keeping the back concave.
3. Slide your hands, palms up, under the sole of the foot and hold for 2 breaths. (Figure 46)
4. EXHALE, bend the elbows and bring the head to the knees.

III. *Dos and Don'ts for the three Forward Bend Variations:*

DO keep the knees absolutely straight and tightened.
DO remember that "concave" means that the back is arched backward.
DO keep the head up while the back is concave.
DO breathe rather deeply.
DO start easy as a beginner with simple forward bending.
DO NOT push or force any position.

People with disc problems must not bring the head to the knees. Each variation is fun to explore but also affects slightly different areas, so that the practice of all is recommended.

*Basic pose described in ABC of Yoga.

Variation 3: (Ardha Baddha Padmottanasana)

1. Stand, the feet together.
2. INHALE, lift the right leg and bring it to above the knee of the left leg.
3. Bend slightly forward and grasp the right ankle with both hands. (Figure 47)
4. *Gently* lift the right foot as high up as possible on the left thigh.
5. EXHALE, bend forward, keeping the back concave, and
6. Put the hands on the floor. If very advanced, bring the right hand behind the back and grasp the toes of the right foot, using only the left hand for support on the floor. (Figure 48 and 49)
7. EXHALE, bring the head to the knee and hold for 10-20 seconds.
8. INHALE, straighten out and relax. Repeat on the other side.

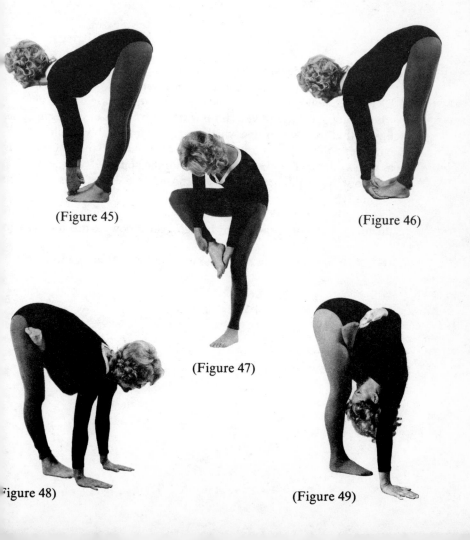

(Figure 45)

(Figure 46)

(Figure 47)

(Figure 48)

(Figure 49)

*FORWARD BEND (SITTING) (PASCHIMOTTANASANA) VARIA-TIONS

I. *Benefits:*

Forward Bend (Sitting) Variations. . .
- strengthen the *abdominal muscles* and tone the *abdominal organs.*
- stretch, limber up and release *tension* in *legs* and *spine.*
- are beneficial to the entire *nervous system.*
- aid *digestion* and *elimination.*
- tone the *kidneys.*
- massage the *heart.*
- stretch the *pelvic region* and improve the *circulation* there.
- give a feeling of *vitality.*

II. *Technique:*

1. Sit on the floor, legs stretched out, feet together and back straight.
2. Raise your arms perpendicular to the legs and lean back slightly.
3. EXHALE, slowly bend forward with a curling motion of the spine and when you have reached your limit without straining or bouncing, grasp tightly that part of your leg which you can comfortably reach.
4. Now bend your elbows and concentrate on pulling your body forward as well as down, to give a good stretch to the spine.
5. Let your head hang and hold the pose for 5-30 seconds, breathing normally.
6. Eventually you will be able to bring your head to your knees and grasp the toes instead of the ankles by bringing the elbows to the floor. (Figure 50)
7. INHALE, return slowly out of the pose and repeat twice more.

*Basic pose described in ABC of Yoga.

Variations-On-a-Theme; for the bored, advanced student:

1. Grasp the big toes between the thumb and the next two fingers, and proceed with Forward Bend, bending the elbows for a good spinal stretch.
2. OR, clasp the fingers around the soles of the feet.
3. OR, clasp the soles of the feet by bringing the wrists over the top of the toes.
4. OR, clasp one wrist with the other hand around the soles of the feet. (Figure 51)

(Figure 50)

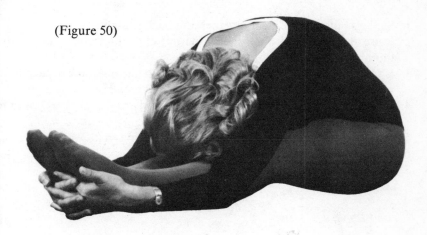

(Figure 51)

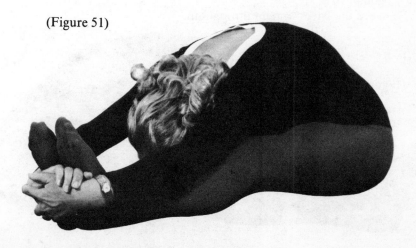

Variation 1: (Parivrtta Paschimottanasana)

I. *Benefits:*

The Twisted Forward Bend . . .
- aids *digestion* and *elimination.*
- relieves *backache* by its lateral twisting action.
- increases *energy* and *vitality* and helps to cure *impotency.*
- tones the *spine* and *kidneys.*

II. *Technique:*

1. Sit, legs outstretched, feet together and back straight.
2. Raise the arms and cross them, the left over the right, pointing the thumbs towards the floor.
3. EXHALE and bend slowly forward grasping the outer sole of each foot, with the arms still crossed. Take two normal breaths.
4. EXHALE, bend the elbows and twist the body to the left, and bringing the head between the arms, look up. (Figure 52)
5. Hold the pose from 10-20 seconds, the breathing shallow.
6. INHALE, straighten the body and relax.
7. Repeat, with the position of the arms reversed.

III. *Dos and Don'ts:*

DO practise the pose as in the Ear to Knee pose at first if you encounter difficulties.

DO bring the right upper arm against the outside of the left knee to insure a good twist.

DO keep the knees straight throughout.

(Figure 52)

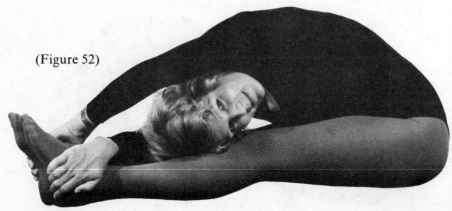

Variation 2: (Urdhva Mukha Paschimottanasana)

I. *Benefits:*

The Intense Forward Bend . . .
- strengthens and firms the *thighs.*
- makes the *calves* shapely.
- relieves even bad *backaches.*
- promotes *balance* and poise and therefore. . .
- corrects *bad posture.*

II. *Technique:*

1. Lie on your back, legs straight, arms stretched back. Take two normal breaths.
2. EXHALE, and slowly raise the legs, pressing the small of the back against the floor—as in the Plough.
3. Clasp the hands and bring them up and around the bottom of the feet, keeping the legs straight, and the whole of the back pressed against the floor. Take two normal breaths. (Figure 53)
4. EXHALE and pull the legs toward the face by bending the elbows.
5. Hold, breathing normally, for 10-60 seconds.
6. INHALE, lower the legs and relax.
7. Repeat, if the pose was not held very long.

III. *Dos and Don'ts:*

DO keep the knees straight.
DO keep the back as close to the floor as possible throughout the exercise.
DO try to bring the legs to the head.
DO NOT raise the head.

(Figure 53)

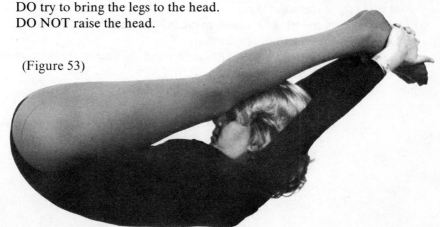

Variation 3: (Triang Mukhaikapada Paschimottanasana)

I. *Benefits:*

The Three-Part Forward Bend ...
- aids *digestion* and *elimination.*
- cures *stiff knees* and *ankles.*
- firms the *abdomen.*
- helps to cure *flat feet.*
- stretches, limbers up and releases *tension* in *legs* and *spine.*

II. *Technique:*

1. Sit in the Sitting Warrior Pose (on your knees, the feet beside the hips.)
2. With the hands by your side shift your weight to the left knee and extend the right leg straight forward.
3. EXHALE, bend slowly forward, sliding the hands down the right leg and grasp the foot.
4. Bend the elbows and with a steady pull stretch back forward rather than down.
5. Let the head hang and attempt to bring the chin to the knee eventually.
6. Hold the pose for 10-30 seconds, breathing normally. (Figure 54)
7. INHALE, straighten up and relax.
8. Repeat with the other leg.

III. *Dos and Don'ts:*
DO keep the right knee straight and tightened.
DO bring the knees together.
DO balance on the left knee, leaning the body slightly in that direction.
DO NOT let the elbows touch the floor.
DO grab one wrist with the other hand around the sole of the foot, as you become more advanced.

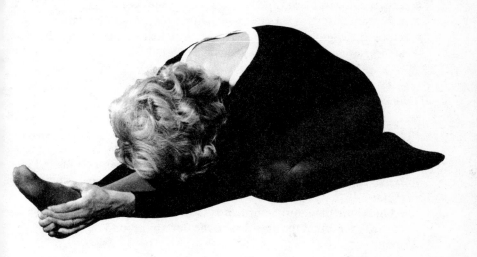

(Figure 54)

All the variations of the Forward Bend combine the basic benefits with the specifically stated ones. Instead of performing the same forward bending pose every day, try out a Variation for every day of the week. They combine a tremendous abdominal massage with a kink-removing stretch of the back, legs and pelvic area. They are for you!

FROG (BHEKASANA)

I. *Benefits:*

The Frog . . .
- relieves *rheumatic* pain in the *knees.*
- massages and stimulates the *abdominal organs.*
- strengthens the *ankles* and relieves *pain.*
- helps to cure *flat feet* through pressure on the arch.
- softens *calcaneal spurs* and relieves *pain* in the *heels.*
- is recommended for *varicose veins,* with a *short* holding motion.
- removes *fatigue* from the *legs* and *feet* (excellent for hairdressers, waitresses and similar professions)

II. *Technique:*

1. Lie on the floor, face down, arms stretched back.
2. Bend the knees and bring the heels close to the buttocks.
3. Place the right hand on the right foot and the left hand on the left one.
4. EXHALE, lift your head and shoulders off the floor, looking up. (Figure 55)
5. At the same time, turn your hands so that the four fingers grasp the top of the foot around the outside and the thumbs around the inside of each foot.
6. Press down on the feet, pushing them towards the floor on each side.
7. Hold the pose from 10-30 seconds, breathing normally. (Figure 56)
8. EXHALE, lower the body and relax.
9. Repeat.

III. *Dos and Don'ts:*

DO be sure to place the hands properly on the feet. The motion is one of pushing down rather than pulling down.

DO prepare for the Frog with such exercises as the Sitting and Reclining Warrior, the Japanese Sitting Position and the Lotus.

DO follow the breathing instructions accurately.

DO NOT force the feet down beyond comfort.

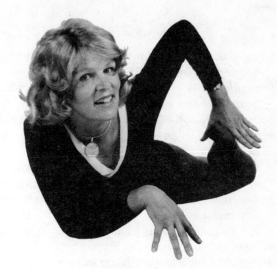

(Figure 55)

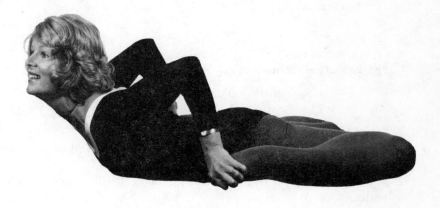

(Figure 56)

The Frog, like the Bow, is a little tricky to perform at first but becomes amazingly simple with proper execution. As an exercise involving the feet and legs it is unsurpassed.

HEADSTAND VARIATIONS (SALAMBA SIRSASANA)

I. *Benefits:*

Headstand Variations . . .
Owing to the reversal of the normal upright position, the following benefits
are derived from the Headstand:
- *circulation* is greatly improved to areas which normally get little: i)
  brain, ii) *heart,* iii) *pelvis,* iv) *spinal cord.*
- the *nervous system* is toned owing to balancing and circulation.
- *abdominal organs,* which normally sag or prolapse, are pulled into
  original position.
- *stomach muscles* are firmed and strengthened.
- *sinus fluids* are now permitted to flow downward.
- the *endocrine, pituitary* and *pineal glands* are stimulated into normal
  action.
- *energy* and a general feeling of *alertness* are experienced.
- strengthens the *lungs.*
- *digestion* and *elimination* are improved.
- the following ailments are removed or their condition is improved:
    - a) insomnia and nerves
    - b) colds and sore throats
    - c) palpitations
    - d) bad breath
    - e) headaches
    - f) asthma
    - g) varicose veins
    - h) lack of sexual interest

II. *Technique:*

1. Make sure that you have adequate support for your head: a carpet with
   underfelt or a blanket folded in four.
2. Kneel on the carpet or in front of the blanket with your toes tucked
   under.
3. Clasp your hands tightly and place them on the floor with the elbows
   not more, nor less, than a shoulder's width apart.
4. Place the very top of the head on the floor, disregarding the hands for
   now.
5. Now pull the folded hands against the back of the head *on the floor.* The
   little fingers will be under the curvature of the head.
6. Push your bottom straight up and with the knees absolutely straight
   throughout, slowly tippy-toe up towards your head. The object is to
   make the back straight. (Figure 57)

7. When you can do so without pushing, gently lift off the toes, bend your knees and bring the heels to the buttocks. EXHALE, and (Figure 58)
8. Balance in this position until you are secure, then *slowly* straighten out the legs.
9. Tuck your bottom in and try to get the body into a completely vertical line. (Figure 59)
10. Hold this position from 10 seconds to 5 minutes, increasing your time by a minute a week or according to your ability.
11. Return the legs *slowly* to the floor by bending the knees and reversing the getting- up process.

(Figure 57)

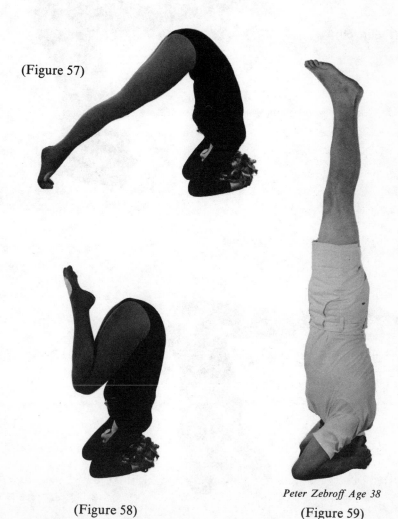

Peter Zebroff Age 38

(Figure 58)   (Figure 59)

Variations-on-a-Theme 1:

1. Follow steps 1-6 and then continue, bringing the legs up, feet together, in a straight line, without bending the knees. Come down the same way. Figure 60)

2. OR, follow steps 1-6, spread the legs apart and raise the legs, knees straight, on the sides, bringing the feet together when the body is in a vertical profile. (Figure 61)

(Figure 60)

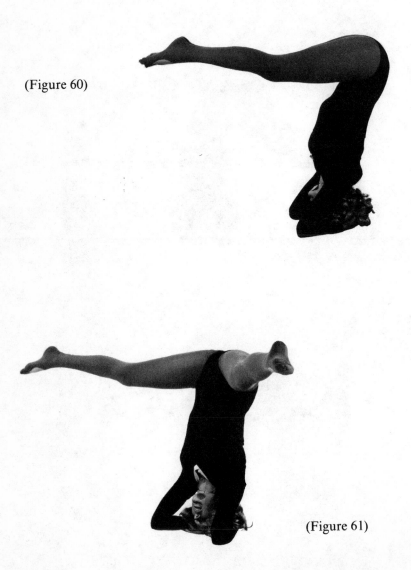

(Figure 61)

Variations -on-a-Theme 2:

When you have achieved perfect balance in the Headstand, assume the
   following leg positions while topsy-turvy.

1. Cross your ankles OR assume an Eagle Position.
2. Spread the legs to the sides.
3. Spread the legs as you would while walking, one leg pointing forward,
   the other pointing back. (Figure 61a)
4. Spread the legs and then twist from the waist, leaving the legs absolutely
   immobile in the hip joints. (Figure 62)
5. Cross the thighs and in this position spread them as far as possible.
   (Figure 63)
6. As above, but with a twist in the waist.
7. Assume the Lotus Position. (Figure 64)
8. Bend the knees and let them hang loosely behind the back, toes
   pointing to the floor, back arched. (Figure 65)
9. Assume a tripod position, the soles of the feet touching, the knees
   sideways in a straight line with the body. (Figure 66)
10. Bring one leg straight down on the side, in line with the body, leaving
    the other up. Repeat on the other side.
11. Bring one leg straight down in front, the toes on the floor in front of the
    face. Leave the other leg pointing up. Repeat on the other side.
12. Twist your body to the side, with the legs together, so that the toes are
    pointing at right angles to the body.
13. Practice any variation you can think of, as long as you adhere to the
    basic Yoga principle of slow movement and a holding position. (Figures
    67, 68, 69)

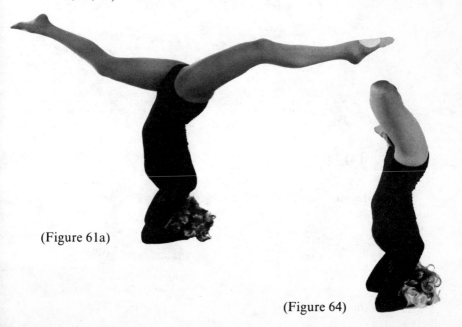

(Figure 61a)

(Figure 64)

70

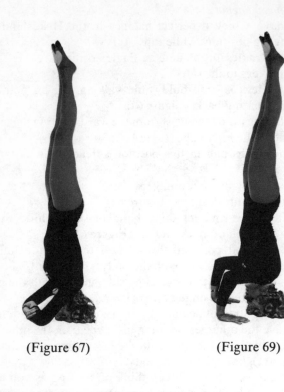

(Figure 67)

(Figure 69)

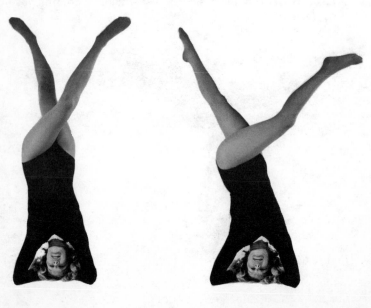

(Figure 63)

(Figure 62)

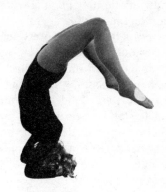

(Figure 65)

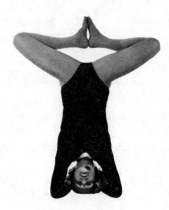

(Figure 66)

The Headstand may be the King of exercises but because it is also an advanced pose, the Shoulderstand may substitute for it for any length of time. Indeed a combination of the two eventually is necessary for greatest health. Familiarize yourself with the Headstand SLOWLY, like forming a life-long friendship —one does not rush that. Find your perfect balance after much experimenting and keep in mind that the head should carry most of the weight, the arms serve as a balance safeguard only. Your pleasure in yourself with the mastery of this pose, and your glowing health will make "SIRSASANA" an indispensable part of your life.

III. *Dos and Don'ts:*

DO clasp your hands very tightly and take your rings off to prevent slipping and undue strain on the arms.

DO NOT let your elbows flare out or press against the head. For a perfect tripod they are a shoulder's width apart.

DO put the crown of the head on the floor. Contrary to what you have learned in calisthenics classes, it is not the hairline nor the back of the head that will support you longest and most comfortably. Eventually you may be able to stand on your head from 5-30 minutes.

DO NOT put the back of the head against the hands but rather bring the hands against the head. Do a little bit of nestling there to make sure you will be comfortable.

DO keep the knees very straight to make possible a straight back.

DO NOT, repeat, DO NOT push up on your toes to get you up into the Headstand. Unless the toes lift off *by themselves* you are not ready to bring the legs up. Even when you are ready, practice balance by hugging the knees to the chest for awhile. The hardest part of the Headstand Proper is bringing the legs up and that is mainly done by strong abdominal muscles. The Headstand is a feat of strength rather than skill.

DO practice the Cobra and the Bow to make the neck strong and flexible. This is especially true for round-shouldered people.

DO practice the Pump, Sit-up and Abdominal Lift to strengthen tummy muscles if you topple over as soon as you try to straighten your legs.

DO practice the balancing position with the knees hugged to the chest, until you can hold it for about a minute before going on with the next steps.

DO or DO NOT (there is a great split in opinion by the experts here) use a corner of the room to practice the Headstand. But if you do, then have the head no further than 2 or 3 inches from the wall, any more would unduly curve the spine and cause pressure on the wrong parts of the body.

DO concentrate fiercely, in order to keep your balance.

DO find a spot or a piece of lint in the carpet and train your eyes on it throughout.

DO practice the Headstand soon after your warm-up while you are still fresh and strong.

DO try to combine the Headstand and Shoulderstand, one after the other in this order, for extra long topsy-turvy benefits.

DO come down just as slowly as you went up.

DO NOT worry if you are not completely straight for awhile; this will come with confidence.

DO tuck your bottom in for a perfect profile.

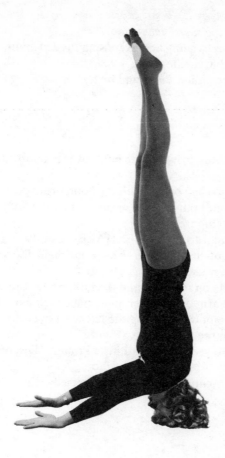

(Figure 68)

DO take your time and be patient with yourself. The Headstand is one of the most difficult poses in Yoga and will take time, strength, flexibility and balance to accomplish. Develop these skills first. The Headstand Attempt will prepare you in all respects for eventually doing the Headstand and it is an excellent exercise in its own right.

HORSE (VATAYANASANA)

I. *Benefits:*

The Horse . . .
- is beneficial to the *sacroiliac* region.
- is excellent for *realigning* and exercising the *hip joints.*
- *strengthens* and firms the *thighs.*
- removes *stiffness* in the *knees* and *ankles.*

II. *Technique:*

1. Sit in a Half-Lotus, bringing the left foot as high up on the right thigh as possible.
2. With your hands by your side on the floor, bring the right foot out from under the left and put the sole of the foot on the floor about 6" in front of the left leg. (Figure 70)
3. Shift your weight to the left, EXHALE, push down on the hands and bring the top of the left knee beside the right foot, straightening the body from the waist.
4. Now, balancing on the knee and the foot, bring your arms forward and cross the right arm over the left one above the elbow.
5. Bend the left elbow and bring the left wrist over the right wrist, palms touching, as in the Eagle Pose. (Figure 71)
6. Hold for 10-30 seconds, breathing normally. Disengage yourself and relax.
7. Repeat, with leg and arm positions reversed.

III. *Dos and Don'ts:*

DO make sure that the left thigh is completely straight—that is, vertical to the floor.

DO concentrate fiercely on your balance.

DO have the arms crossing in the reverse of the legs.

The Horse is not one of the more mandatory of the Yoga postures. However, for the advanced student, or the person with an aching sacroiliac, it paves the way for a truly limber body.

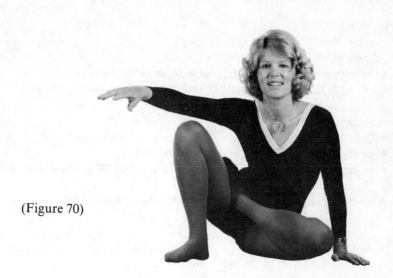

(Figure 70)

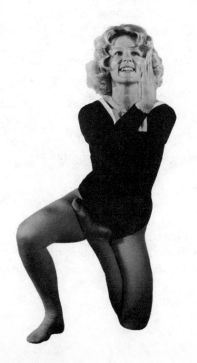

(Figure 71)

INCLINED PLANE (PURVOTTANASANA)

I. *Benefits:*

Inclined Plane . . .
- develops and firms the *pectoral muscles* of the bustline.
- expands the *chest* for easier breathing with *respiratory problems.*
- tightens and firms the *buttocks.*
- strengthens the *wrists.*
- "oils" the shoulder joints.
- strengthens *ankles* and makes them shapely.
- is recommended to offset the forward bending exercises and the shoulderstand.
- Variation 1 is a specific for firming the *hips, thighs,* and *abdomen.*

II. *Technique:*

1. Sit, legs together and outstretched.
2. Lean back slightly and place the hands straight down from the shoulders, fingers pointing forward on the floor. EXHALE, push down on the hands and lift the buttocks off the floor. (Figure 72)
3. Dig the heels in and push the hips up as much as possible, arching the back. Let the head fall back. (Figure 73)
4. Hold for 10-60 seconds breathing normally, letting the hands and feet carry the weight.
5. EXHALE, lower the hips to the floor and relax.

Variation 1:
1. Repeat steps 1-3 as above.
4. Slowly raise the right leg as high as it will go. (Figure 74)
5. Hold for 10-30 seconds.
6. Repeat on the other side.

Variation 2:
1. Sit with legs outstretched, feet together.
2. Put the hands beside the hips with the fingers pointing *backward.*
3. EXHALE, push down on the hands and raise the buttocks off the floor.
4. Proceed with steps 3-5 of Inclined Plane.

The Inclined Plane should always follow forward bending poses, but it is an excellent 'firmer" on its own.

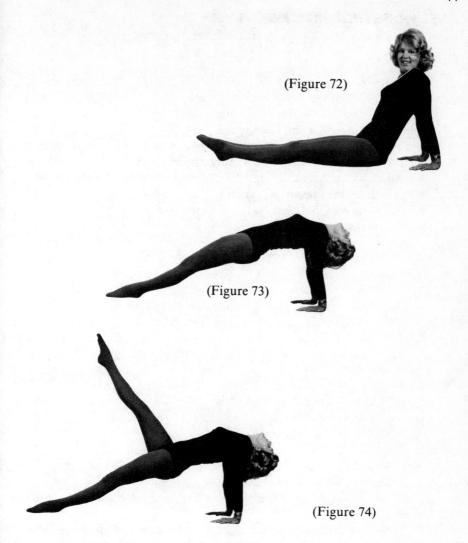

(Figure 72)

(Figure 73)

(Figure 74)

III. *Dos and Don'ts:*

DO bend the knees and bring the soles of the feet flat to the floor, to help you get the buttocks raised, at first. When the pose is achieved straighten the legs.

DO make sure that the whole sole of the foot is resting on the floor, once the pose is achieved.

DO concentrate on the benefits, not the difficulties of the pose, while holding it.

DO distribute the body weight evenly between the hands and feet.

DO stretch the neck back as much as possible, letting the head hang.

KNEE PRESS (WIND-RELIEVING POSE)

I. *Benefits:*

The Knee Press. . .
- is aptly named the *"wind-relieving"* pose.
- relieves *flatulence* and *stomach gas.*
- improves *digestion* and *elimination.*
- is recommended for the greatly *over-weight* and very *elderly,* because it gives maximum results with a minimum of effort.
- relieves *backache* and strengthens the *lumbar* region of the *back.*
- strengthens the *abdominal muscles.*
- eases *tension* in the *neck, back* and *shoulders.*
- strengthens the *neck muscles.*

II. *Technique:*

1. Lie on your back, legs outstretched, hands by your side.
2. Bend the right knee and bring it against the chest.
3. INHALE, clasp your hands around the knee and press it against the abdomen and chest. Keep the left leg straight and the head on the floor.
4. Hold the pose and your breath for 5-10 seconds. (Figure 75)
5. EXHALE, lower the leg and relax.
6. Repeat with the other leg.
7. Repeat with both legs together.

Variation 1:
1. Repeat steps 1 and 2 as above.
3. INHALE, clasp your hands around the right knee and press it to the chest.
4. At the same time bring the head up and try to press it to the knee.
5. Hold the pose and your breath for 5-10 seconds. (Figure 76)
6. EXHALE, lower the leg and relax.
7. Repeat on the other side.
8. Repeat with both knees.

Variation 2:
1. Perform a Sit-Up by lying on your back, placing the hands on the thighs and leaving the legs outstretched. INHALE, slowly lift your head and shoulders as high as you can but do not lift the back. Hold your breath for as long as you can. EXHALE, relax. (Figure 77)
2. As above, but with the legs 3″ off the floor.
3. As above, but with the hands clasped behind the head. (Figure 78)

III. *Dos and Don'ts*

DO NOT hold your breath if you have a record of high blood pressure or heart trouble. Simply inhale and then breathe normally.

DO keep the knee of the out-stretched leg straight.

DO get a good grasp on the knees and exert as much pressure as you can on the abdomen.

DO NOT get discouraged if your knee is nowhere near your head at first. The mere effort does wonders for you.

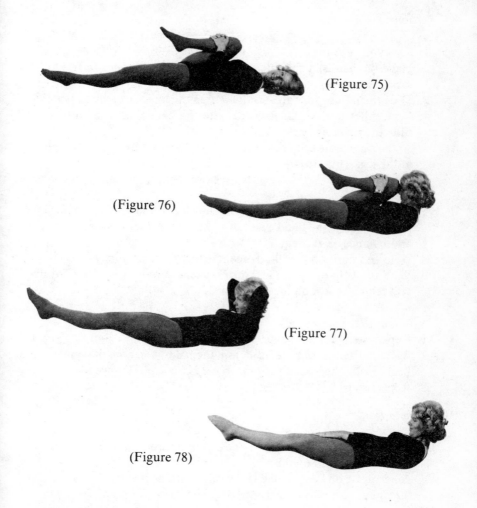

(Figure 75)

(Figure 76)

(Figure 77)

(Figure 78)

The Knee Press is a "NOW" sort of exercise, to be done anytime there is a need for it. It relieves, as well as strengthens.

LEG SPLIT (HANUMANASANA or ANYANEYASANA)

I. *Benefits:*

The Leg Split. . .
- helps to cure *sciatica.*
- tones and makes shapely the whole *leg.*
- firms and strengthens the *thigh.*
- exercises the *hip joint.*
- promotes dancer's *flexibility* and *poise.*

II. *Technique:* Basic Pose

1. Squat on your toes.
2. Place the hands, a shoulder's width apart, on the floor in front of the toes. (Figure 79)
3. Slide the left leg forward, straightening the knee as much as possible.
4. Now shift your weight forward onto the hands, lift the buttocks and slide the right leg backward.
5. At the same time keep sliding the left leg forward to make a straight line of the legs. (Figure 80)
6. Press the groin slowly towards the floor, letting the hands take most of the weight.
7. Once you can sit completely on the floor (and this will take much practice), raise the hands, and bring them together in front of the chest and balance on the legs.
8. Hold this position for 10-30 seconds, breathing normally.
9. With the help of the hands, return to the squatting position, sit down and relax. Repeat on the other side.

Variation: (Very advanced)
1. Repeat steps 1-6 as above.
7. Raise the hands over the head, join the palms and arch the spine up and back. Hold, then bend forward towards the feet. (Figure 81)
8. Repeat steps 8 and 9 as above.

III. *Dos and Don'ts:*

DO NOT, repeat DO NOT, force the groin towards the floor. Let time and your body weight do the work.

DO concentrate on keeping the legs straight, the heel of the forward leg and the upper part of the backward foot resting on the floor.

DO let your hands support your weight at first, only gradually settling on the groin.

DO try the Leg Split out of a Deep Lunge position, if you have difficulty doing it this way.

Most people are familiar with the Leg Split as a ballet position. Please remember that it has taken years of intensive study for the ballerinas to accomplish it and do not be disappointed or force the pose. Just the attempt will vigorously exercise the whole leg.

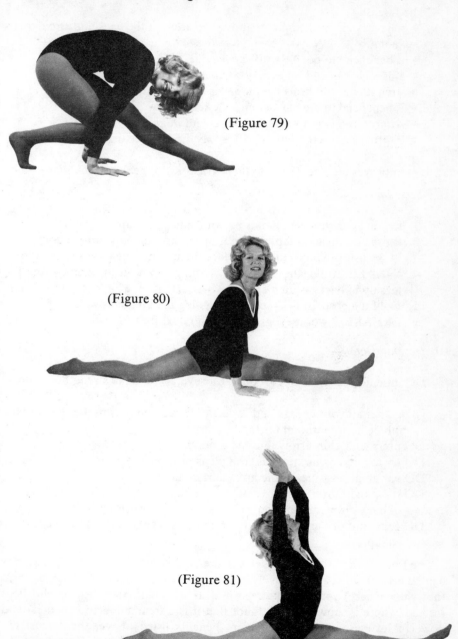

(Figure 79)

(Figure 80)

(Figure 81)

*LOCUST (SALABHASANA)

I. *Benefits:*

The Locust. . .
- relieves pain in the *lumbar* and *sacral* areas of the *back* and strengthens them.
- is beneficial to people with *slipped disc.*
- aids *digestion* and relieves *abdominal complaints.*
- strengthens and firms the *buttocks, abdomen* and *thighs.*
- is beneficial to the *bladder* and the *sex glands.*
- *reduces weight* in the *hips, buttocks* and *thighs.*
- improves the circulation to the *head* for a feeling of *alertness* and *energy.*
- improves the circulation to the *pelvic area* for healthy *glandular action.*

II. *Technique:*

1. Lie on your stomach, hands by your side palms up.
2. Raise your head and place the front of the chin only, on the floor.
3. Make fists of your hands and place them under the thighs in the groin.
4. INHALE, stiffen the body and pushing down on the arms, bring the legs up in back, as high as they will go. (Figures 82 and 83)
5. Hold the pose for 5-10 seconds, holding the breath as well.
6. EXHALE, lower the legs slowly and relax. Rest for awhile.

III. *Dos and Don'ts:*

DO practice the Half-Locust only, for several weeks, to strengthen a weak back.

DO gather all your energy and concentration on your arms and legs as you inhale in preparation for the Locust.

DO press your chin firmly into the ground.

DO try to make your knees as straight as possible.

DO use great pressure on the arms to raise the legs.

DO try a slight thrusting movement to get the legs up, *if* you have no record of back problems, and only after a thorough warm-up.

DO come out of the pose slowly. You nullify a great deal of your effort by collapsing.

The Locust is a pose of controversy in the Yoga source books. Since it requires a great deal of effort and relatively sudden movement in its very advanced form (not shown here) some books regard it as un-Yogic and support the Boat instead. There is, however, no doubt that it is a tremendously beneficial and powerful exercise. Besides the many benefits listed above, the Locust encourages self-discipline and brings to your head a blush not only of improved circulation but one of pride as well.

Variation 1:
1. Proceed with steps 1 and 2, as above.
3. Place the hands, palms up, fingers pointing toward the feet, under the thighs.
4. Proceed with steps 4-6 as above.

Variation 2: The Half-Locust
1. Lie on your stomach, hands by your side, palms up.
2. Make a fist and bring it close to the body.
3. Raise your head and bring the front of the chin to the floor.
4. Pressing the arms against the floor, INHALE and slowly raise the right leg straight up in the back as far as you can. (Figure 84)
5. Hold the breath and the pose from 5-10 seconds, EXHALE and slowly lower the leg. Relax.
6. Repeat on the other side, making sure that the body weight is not rolled to the side of the out-stretched leg.
7. As a variation you may make the fists and place them *thumbs* down.

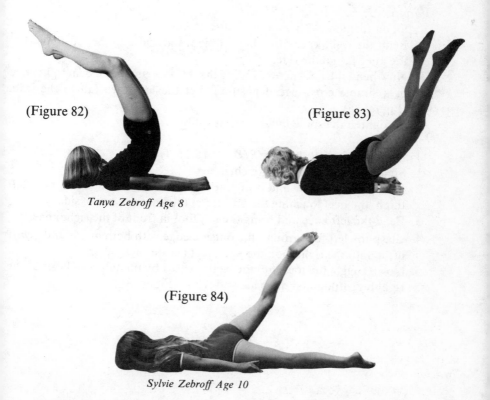

(Figure 82)

(Figure 83)

Tanya Zebroff Age 8

(Figure 84)

Sylvie Zebroff Age 10

*Look for *Boat* in ABC of Yoga for a variation of the pose.

THE LOTUS (PADMASANA)

I. *Benefits:*

The Lotus. . .
- encourages a good natural curve of the *spine* and thereby improves *posture.*
- lowers the body metabolism if practiced for any length of time and therefore is very *restful physically* and wonderfully *relaxing mentally.*
- enhances the power of *concentration* and mental *alertness.*
- tones the *abdominal organs.*
- limbers up the *ankles* and *knees.*
- tones the *spine.*
- is recommended for *meditation* and *breath control.*

II. *Technique:* The following poses should be mastered before a complete Lotus (very advanced) is attempted.

Variation 1: Easy Posture (SUKHASANA)
1. Sit on the floor with your legs outstretched.
2. Bend the right knee, bringing the right foot close to the left thigh. Let the knee fall to the side.
3. Now bend the left knee and bring the left foot under the bent right knee in a simple cross-legged position. Let the left knee fall to the side. (Figure 85)
4. Straighten the spine but do not sit stiffly.

*Variation 2: Perfect Posture (SIDDHASANA)
1. Sit on the floor, legs outstretched.
2. Bend the right knee and bring the right sole of the foot against the left thigh, the heel touching the groin. Let the knee fall to the side.
3. Bend the left knee and bring the left foot in front of the right knee.
4. Clasp the left foot around the outside edge with both hands and *gently* lift it onto the right foot, the heels just beside each other.
5. Now snuggle the toes into the cleft created by the thigh and calf of the right leg. Straighten the back and relax. (Figure 86)

*See complete description in ABC of Yoga.

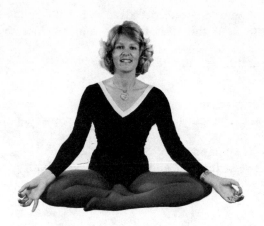

(Figure 85)

(Figure 86)

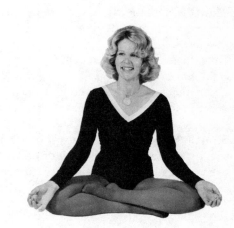

86

Variation 3: Half Lotus

1. Repeat steps 1-3 as above.
4. Clasp the left foot, around the outside edge, with both hands and *gently* lift it onto the right thigh, as high up and as close to the groin as possible.
5. Straighten the spine and relax. (Figure 87)

Variation 4: Ankle-Lock (SWASTIKASANA)

1. Sit on the floor, legs outstretched.
2. Bend the right knee and bring the heel against the groin, placing the *top* of the foot against the thigh.
3. Repeat steps 3 and 4 of Variation 1.
4. Tuck the toes in between the calf and the thigh. Now both feet are placed this way, one with the toes up, the other with toes down. (Figure 88)
6. Straighten the spine and relax.

Variation 5: Full Lotus (PADMASANA)

1. Sit on the floor, legs outstretched.
2. Bend the right knee, letting it fall to the side, and bring the sole of the right foot to the left thigh.
3. Clasp the right foot around the outside edge with both hands and gently place it onto the left thigh as high up and as close to the groin as possible.
4. Now bend the left knee and bring the left foot in front of the right knee.
5. Clasp the left foot around the outside edge with both hands and gently lift it onto the right thigh, as high up and as close to the groin as possible.
6. Straighten the spine and place your hands, palms up, on each knee. Join the tips of the thumbs to the index fingers. Relax. Close your eyes. You are now ready for meditation. (Figure 89)

III. *Dos and Don'ts:*

DO make very sure that the head, neck and back are in a straight line while sitting in any of the above positions.

DO wear tights or similar apparel at the beginning. There is a tension created by the toes slipping off the thighs that may be painful on the bare leg.

DO NOT repeat DO NOT, in any way force a Lotus position. The knee is easily twisted.

DO let your knees fall to the side, and practice such exercises as the Knee & Thigh Stretch to limber up.

DO bring your heels as close to the perineum (the exact centre of the body) as possible.

DO NOT get discouraged if your knees stick up like craggy twin mountains at first. It is regular practice that brings results.

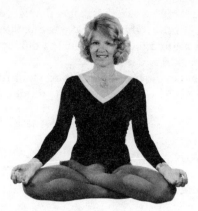

(Figure 87)

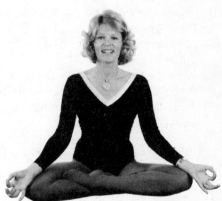

(Figure 88)

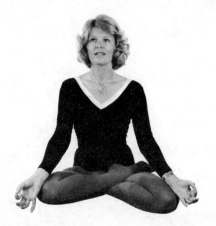

(Figure 89)

Variation 6: Bound Lotus (BADDHA PADMASANA)

1. Sit in a full Lotus with the right leg on top.
2. EXHALE and, knifing the shoulder blades together, bring the right arm around the back catching the toes of the right foot. Take two breaths.
3. EXHALE and bring the left arm around the back, catching the toes of the left foot. Let the head hang back. Take two breaths.
4. EXHALE and bend forward bringing the head to the floor. Hold 10-60 seconds, breathing normally. EXHALE, straighten out, unfold and relax.
5. As a variation of this, bend forward to either knee in turn. (Figure 90)

Variation 7: Sense Sealer (SANMUKHI MUDRASANA)

1. Sit in a full erect Lotus.
2. Bend your elbows and bring them up on the sides, the hands on the face.
3. Close your eyes and place the first two fingers on the eyelids.
4. Place the third (ring) fingers against the nostrils narrowing the breathing channel but not closing it off. The little fingers are on the upper lip.
5. Press the thumbs against the ears. (Figure 91)
6. Breathe evenly and deeply for as long as you can. This pose is excellent for reducing tension or mental turmoil. Peace pervades the whole body and meditation is a natural conclusion.

Variation 8: Symbol of Yoga (YOGA MUDRA)

1. Sit in a full Lotus.
2. Bring the arms around the back, clasping one wrist with the other hand.
3. INHALE deeply and as you exhale, bend forward, touching your head to the floor. (Figure 92)
4. Hold, breathing normally, for as long as you can. EXHALE, straighten up, unfold and relax.

The Lotus position is a very advanced one and often takes years to accomplish. Maddeningly, however, some people can do it almost immediately, even if they are not particularly flexible otherwise. Any of the simple poses mentioned above will do very nicely for the beginner in meditation and breath control.

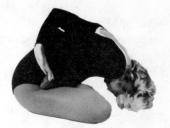

(Figure 90)

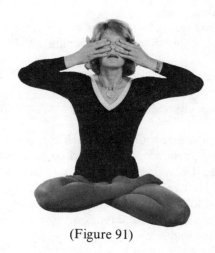

(Figure 91)

(Figure 92)

MARICHI'S POSE (MARICHYASANA)

I. *Benefits:*

The Pose of Marichi. . .
- promotes good *circulation* to the abdominal organs.
- improves *digestion.*
- is beneficial to the *dorsal part* of the back.
- strengthens *fingers.*

II. *Technique:*

1. Sit with the legs extended, spine straight.
2. Bend the left knee and place the whole sole of the foot on the floor beside the knee.
3. Now bring the foot up, bringing the heel as close to the body as possible. The calf and thigh should be touching and the knee should point straight up.
4. Extend the left arm and bend slightly forward, bringing the left armpit against the front of the knee. (Figure 93)
5. Now bend the elbow back and wrap the arm around the knee, palm facing up.
6. Bring the arm as far around your back as is possible.
7. Move the right arm around the back as well, attempting to have the fingers touch. If advanced, clasp wrists. (Figure 94)
8. Twist slightly left and look at the right toe. Hold, for 3 breaths.
9. Exhale, bend forward and attempt to put either the chin, lips, nose or forehead to the knee. Hold, breathing normally. (Figure 95)
10. Inhale, unwind and relax.
11. Repeat on the other side.

III. *Dos and Don'ts:*

DO keep the foot touching the right thigh.
DO NOT let the knee fall to the side—it makes wrapping the arm around it more difficult.
DO bend forward enough to get the arm pit, rather than the side of the arm around the knee.
DO NOT get discouraged if your head is nowhere near your right knee at first. That takes quite a while in this pose.

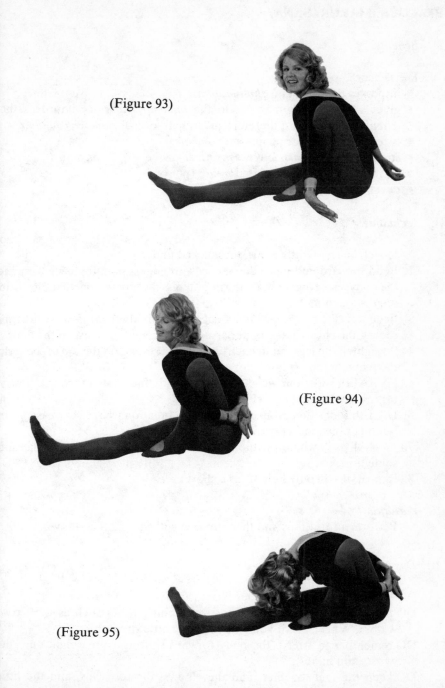

(Figure 93)

(Figure 94)

(Figure 95)

Marichi's Pose is an excellent preparation for any forward bend. These, in turn, are specifics for keeping the abdomen and its organs healthy and firm.

PEACOCK (MAYURASANA)

I. *Benefits:*

The Peacock. . .
- improves *digestion* and *elimination.*
- gives a marvellous massage to the *abdominal organs,* improves the *circulation* there and therefore *relieves* all sorts of *stomach complaints.*
- is recommended for people with *diabetes.*
- strengthens the *wrist, lower arm* and *elbows.*
- rids the body of accumulated *toxins* (poisons).
- develops *arms* and *shoulders.*

II. *Technique:*

1. Kneel, knees slightly apart, toes tucked under.
2. Bend forward and place the hands, with fingers pointing back towards the body, close together, on the floor. Press the elbows together, the little fingers touching.
3. Bend the elbows and press them against the body (near the diaphragm) resting the chest on the upper arms. The face will be close to the floor.
4. Straighten the legs out in back one by one, resting on the top of the feet, the feet together. (Figure 96)
5. EXHALE, shift your weight onto the hands and stretch forward, slowly raising the legs in back. (Figure 97)
6. Hold this position from 5-30 seconds, breathing hard. Increase your holding time gradually over a matter of weeks.
7. EXHALE, slowly lower the body to the floor, head first and relax for some time.
8. Repeat, if you only hold it for a short time.

Variation 1:
Perform a full Lotus and then proceed with steps 2-8 as above.

III. *Dos and Don'ts:*

DO use a pillow in front of your face to give you confidence at first.
DO practice other wrist and arm-strengthening poses such as the Crow, Cobra, Wheel, etc. if you find you have little strength.
DO remember to stretch the body forward shifting your weight onto the wrists and hands.
DO keep the feet together, and the elbows, the forearms, and the little fingers touching.
DO as a woman, try the pose without a bra, arranging the breasts for least pressure.

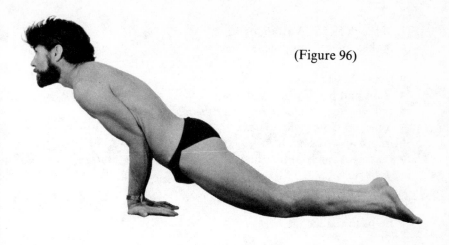

(Figure 96)

Duncan McDougall Age 42

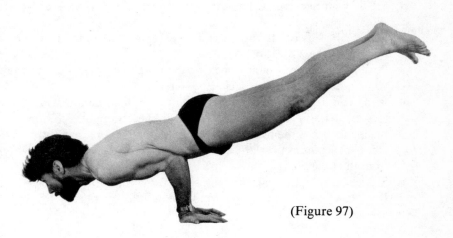

(Figure 97)

    The Peacock is a real HE-MAN pose and not necessary nor recommended for the ladies to accomplish. For the men, it is often easier than it looks at first. "Hurrah" for a pose that is fun to do, looks most impressive and gives tremendous health benefits.

*PLOUGH VARIATIONS (HALASANA)

I. *Benefits:*

The Plough and its Variations. . .
- makes the *spine* supple.
- stimulates the *thyroid gland* for weight control.
- strengthens and firms the *abdomen.*
- slims and firms *thighs* and *hips.*
- relieves deep-seated *tension* and *headaches.*
- tones up the *nervous system.*
- improves *circulation.*
- massages such abdominal organs as the *liver, spleen, pancreas* and *kidneys.*
- acts as an *energy* pick-me-up.
- strengthens the *neck.*
- helps to reduce the *bust.*

II. *Technique:*

Variation 1:
1. Lie on your back on the floor, legs outstretched, arms extended by your side, palms down.
2. EXHALE, slowly lift your legs by tightening the abdominal and leg muscles. Take 2 breaths.
3. Push down on your hands, making them hollow or tent-like and raise your buttocks and lower back. EXHALE.
4. Bring your legs over your head, and touch the floor behind you with the toes, by bending at the waist. Keep your knees straight.
5. Place the top of the feet on the floor, tighten the knees and stretch the feet back as far as possible. The back should be completely straight up from the floor.
6. Stretch your hands, palms down, away from you. (Figure 98)
7. Hold 10-60 seconds, working up to five minutes eventually.

*Basic pose is described in ABC of Yoga.

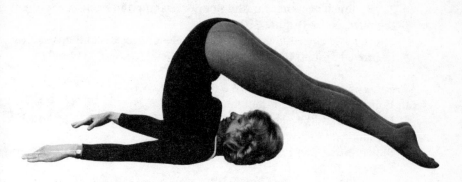

(Figure 98)

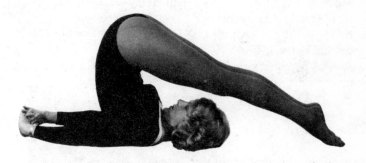

(Figure 99)

Variations-On-A-Theme:
1. Follow steps 1-7 as above.
8. Now bend the elbows, bring the hands up slightly and lock the thumbs. Lower the hands and stretch the arms.
9. As a variation clasp the hands, and turn the wrists until the thumbs are on the floor, the palms away from the body. (Figure 99)

Variation 2: Ear Presser (KARNAPIDASANA)

1. Follow steps 1-6 as in the Plough above.
7. Now bend and spread the knees and bring them down beside the ears. Try to touch the knees to the floor, stretching the back. Keep the feet together. Hold. (Figure 100)
   Special Benefits: the heart and the legs are rested, the circulation is improved around the waistline.

Variation 3: Spreading Plough (SUPTA KONASANA)

1. Follow steps 1-6 as in the Plough.
7. Now spread the legs as far apart as possible, the toes touching the floor.
8. Slowly bring the arms to the toes in a wide circling motion and grasp them. Hold. (Figure 101)
   Special Benefits: the abdominal organs are contracted, the legs are toned.

Variation 4: The Lateral Plough (PARSVA HALASANA)

1. Follow steps 1-6 as in the Plough.
7. Bring your hands against the back for support and to make the back straighter.
8. Move both the legs, knees straight, as far to the right as possible, the toes on the floor. (Figure 102)
9. Hold for 10-30 seconds, EXHALE and move the legs to the left, stretching them. Hold 10-30 seconds.
   Special Benefits: Constipation, and the side-effects deriving from it, are alleviated.

III. *Dos and Don'ts:*

DO keep your knees straight throughout.
DO breathe normally.
DO NOT lift your head as you lower your legs.
DO stretch the arms and the legs away from the trunk.
DO use the hands to straighten the back farther, then bring them back to the
   suggested position.

The Plough is an exercise you will *want* to do once you have mastered its basic position. It is such a pleasure to do that one could easily forget the tension reducing stretch it gives to an unnaturally compressed spine.

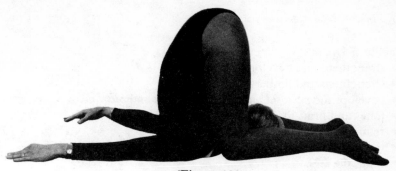

(Figure 100)

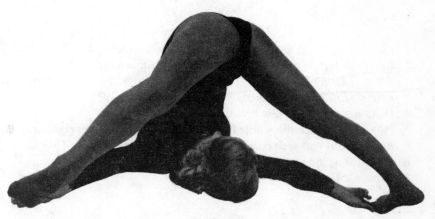

(Figure 101)

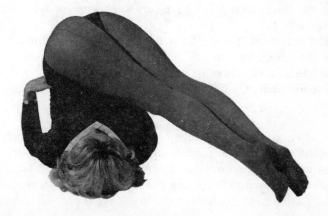

(Figure 102)

PUSH-UP (CHATURANGA DANDASANA)

I. *Benefits:*

The Push-Up. . .
- strengthens and develops the *arms.*
- strengthens and limbers up the *wrists.*
- develops the *pectoral muscles* of the *chest* and *bustline.*
- tones and firms the *abdominal organs.*
- reduces tension in the *toes.*
- tightens the *buttocks.*
- tones the *legs.*
- fills out and develops the *upper arm.*

II. *Technique:*

1. Lie face down on your stomach, toes tucked under.
2. Bring the hands beside the chest, fingers pointing forward.
3. EXHALE, push down on the hands and raise the whole body *in a straight line* a few inches above the floor. (Figure 103)
4. Hold the pose for a few breaths.
5. Now slowly slide the whole body forward, shifting the weight onto the hands, until you are resting on the top of the feet. (Figure 104)
6. Hold for as long as you can or 10-30 seconds.
7. Slowly lower the body and relax.

III. *Dos and Don'ts:*

DO practice this posture if you have very weak wrists or to fill out the upper arm.

DO make very sure that the body is ram rod straight throughout. Ask a friend to check for you.

DO NOT tense up but breathe normally.

DO try to distribute the weight equally between the four points of contact.

The Push-Up may properly be called one of those specifically male exercises. However, if the wrists need strengthening, the bustline needs filling out or the upper arms are discouragingly skinny, regular practice of the Push-Up is recommended. Simply stop practicing it when you have achieved the desired results! And, having tried it, who dares to say, Yoga is only for women?

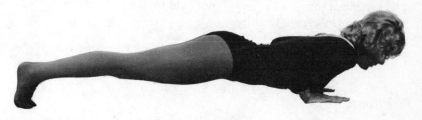

(Figure 103)

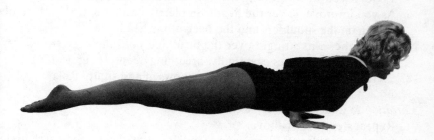

(Figure 104)

RECLINING WARRIOR (SUPTA VIRASANA)

I. *Benefits:*

The Reclining Warrior. . .
* tones and stretches the *abdominal* and *pelvic area.*
* eases *breathing* for *asthma* sufferers.
* stretches and makes shapely the *thighs* and *legs.*
* relieves *aching legs* if done for ten minutes.
* is beneficial for *varicose veins* if not held for long.
* keeps *genital organs* healthy.
* is beneficial for *flat feet.*
* relieves *rheumatic pain* in the *knees* and *heels.*

II. *Technique:*

1. Kneel in an upright position, knees together, the feet a foot and a half apart.
2. Slowly lower your body to sit between the feet *on the floor.* Use your hands for support if you wish.
3. Straighten your back and keep the toes pointed straight back. (Figure 105)
4. EXHALE, lean back and bring your elbows to the floor one by one.
5. Let your head hang back and slowly straighten the arms (clasping the ankles if you wish), shifting the weight onto the top of the head.
6. As you improve, lower the head completely until you are comfortably resting on the shoulders and the back of the head.
7. Stretch the arms straight over the head and hold the pose from a few seconds to 10 minutes eventually, breathing deeply. (Figure 106)
8. EXHALE, grab the ankles, dig the elbows in and sit up. Relax.

Variation 1: Couch (PARYANKASANA)
1. Repeat steps 1-5 as above.
6. Grasp the ankles and give a gentle pull forward to get a good arch in the back.
7. Bring both arms up and clasp the forearms near the elbows. Place the folded arms over the head and try to touch the floor.
8. Hold 10-60 seconds breathing normally.
9. INHALE, clasp the ankles, dig the elbows in and sit up. Relax.
    Special Benefits of the Couch: a regulating of the thyroid gland for weight control (overweight and underweight), easier breathing for respiratory problems.

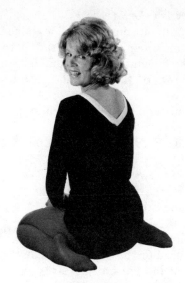

(Figure 105)

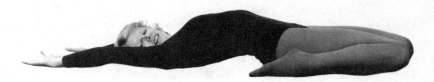

(Figure 106)

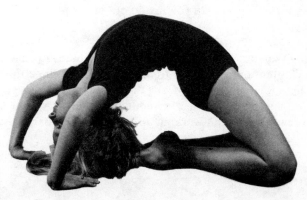

(Figure 107)

Variation 2: Pigeon (KAPOTASANA)
1. Repeat steps 1-6 of the Reclining Warrior above.
7. Now bring the arms up and over the head, placing them on the floor beside the ears, the fingers pointing to the shoulders (as in the wheel).
8. EXHALE, push down on the hands and push the hips up, arching the back.
9. Straighten the arms and thighs as much as possible, contracting the buttocks.
10. Hold 10-30 seconds, EXHALE and lower the body. Relax.

Variation 3: Pigeon (Very advanced)
1. Follow steps 1-4 of Reclining Warrior.
5. Now, stretch up and bring the hands to the toes, resting the elbows on the floor.
6. Take several breaths, EXHALE and grasping the heels attempt to bring the crown of the head on the soles of the feet. (Figure 107)
Special Benefits of the Pigeon: massages and strengthens the heart, develops the chest and bustline, strengthens and firms the abdomen and thighs.

III. *Dos and Don'ts:*

DO NOT force the Reclining Warrior position without being comfortable in the Sitting Warrior first.
DO keep the knees apart at first, to permit full execution of the pose.
DO just place the hands beside the thighs if stretching them over the head proves difficult.
DO take your time (a matter of weeks, if necessary) in bringing the head from a top of the head to a back of the head position.
DO practice this pose instead of the Fish-in-the-Lotus position for the same benefits.
DO grasp your ankles to help you in and out of the pose.

The Reclining Warrior is a delightful position to assume after a long, hard day on your feet. The tension just seems to drain out of the fingertips and knees. Stretching, after all, is the basis of all Yoga and this asana gives you the sensation of the spectacular Wheel without its strain. Try it every evening, starting with a few seconds and working up to 10 minutes gradually.

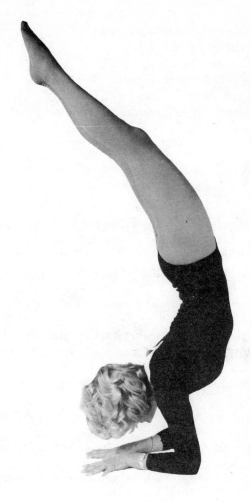

(Figure 108)

The Scorpion depends a great deal on the strength in the arms and is also considered a man's exercise. With concentration and determination, however, many ladies have achieved it, if only for 10 seconds. It is an excellent incentive to continual growth and development in Yoga.

SCORPION (PINCHA MAYURASANA AND VRSCHIKASANA)

I. *Benefits:*

The Scorpion. . .
- stretches and firms the *abdominal muscles.*
- tones and limbers up the *spine.*
- develops *shoulder* and *back muscles.*
- improves *balance* and *coordination.*
- expands the *lungs.*
- improves the *circulation* to the *head, spine* and *pelvic areas.*

II. *Technique:*

Dancing Scorpion (PINCHA MAYURASANA)
1. Kneel on the floor, the toes tucked under.
2. Bend forward and place the forearms on the floor, palms down. The arms should be slightly less than a shoulder's width apart, the fingers are spread apart. (Figure 109)
3. Push down on the feet and bring the bottom up. Raise the head as much as possible.
4. EXHALE, give a slight push with one foot and swing the legs up as in a conventional Handstand.
5. Find your balance by tightening the leg and hip muscles and by stretching the spine, chest and shoulders up. Keep the feet together. (Figure 108)
6. Hold the pose as long as possible, bring the legs down and relax.

Variation 1: Resting Scorpion (SAYANASANA) (Very Advanced)
1. Follow steps 1-6 as above.
7. When you can balance in this pose for at least 20 seconds, bring the hands up one by one, balancing on the elbows.
8. Cup the hands, the wrists touching, and place them under the chin.

Variation 2: Scorpion (VRSCHIKASANA) (Very, very advanced)
1. Follow steps 1-6 as above.
7. EXHALE, arch the back, bring the head up and, bending the knees, attempt to bring the toes to the head. (Figure 110)

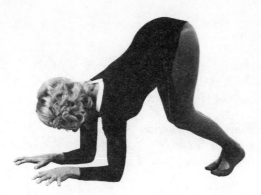

(Figure 109)

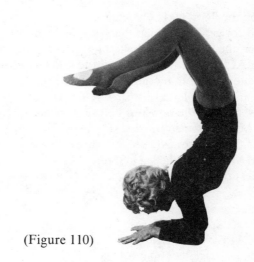

(Figure 110)

III. *Dos and Don'ts:*

DO spread the fingers and slightly "dig in" with the fingertips while balancing in the pose.

DO find the proper spacing of the arms by experimenting. Less than a shoulder's width seems best.

DO practice the pose with the fingertips about a foot from the wall, until you can balance for some time without support.

DO use a slight "springing" action with the shoulders to keep your balance in check at first. (The face might come close to the floor for a moment while you regain your balance).

DO Practice a Handstand first if you think it easier.

DO keep the head up, and the whole body stretched as though someone was pulling up on your toes.

SHOOTING BOW POSE (AKARNA DHANURASANA)

I. *Benefits:*

The Shooting Bow. . .
- limbers up the *hip joints.*
- exercises and makes the *legs* shapely.
- gives a good workout to the *lower spine.*
- aids in *elimination.*
- tones the muscles of *arms* and *shoulders.*
- firms the *thighs* and *hips.*

II. *Technique:*

1. Sit on the floor, legs outstretched.
2. Bend forward and grasp the right toe with the right thumb and index finger, the left toe with the left fingers. (Figure 111)
3. EXHALE, bend the right knee, and pull the right foot towards the right ear in one smooth motion, bringing the right shoulder back.
4. Visualize your leg as the arrow that is being pulled back against the drawstring of the bow just before its release. Keep hold of the left leg and keep the knee straight. (Figure 112)
5. Hold the pose for 5-15 seconds, breathing normally.
6. EXHALE, lower the leg and relax.
7. Repeat on the other side.

Variation 1:
1. Follow steps 1-5 as above.
6. EXHALE and straighten the right knee perpendicular to the floor as much as possible. (Figure 113)
7. Hold 5-15 seconds, breathing normally.
8. EXHALE, lower the leg and relax.

Variation 2:
1. Sit on the floor, the legs outstretched.
2. Bend forward and grasp the right big toe with the thumb and index finger of the left hand.
3. EXHALE, bend the right leg and bring the right foot over the left knee. Take two normal breaths, and. . .
4. Grasp the left big toe with the right hand. Keep the left leg straight.
5. EXHALE and pull the right foot towards the left ear. (Figure 114)
6. Hold for 5-15 seconds, breathing normally.
7. EXHALE and repeat on the other side.

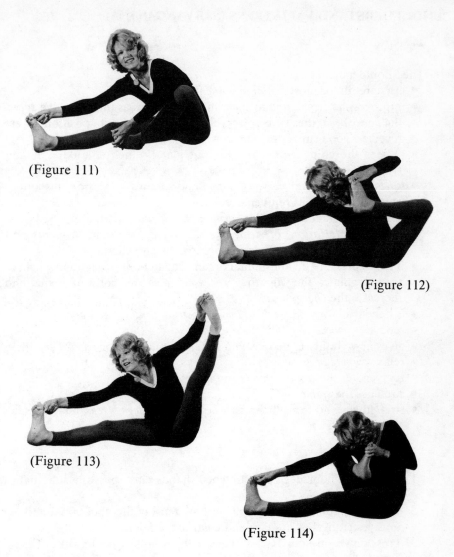

(Figure 111)

(Figure 112)

(Figure 113)

(Figure 114)

III. *Dos and Don'ts:*

    DO keep the knee of the outstretched leg straight and touching the floor.
    DO get a good grip on the foot, grasping all the toes with all the fingers if you wish.
    DO bend forward to meet the foot at first and gradually straighten the back.

    The Shooting Bow Pose takes some practice until good balance is mastered but amongst other things the creaks are taken out of the hip area and that makes it worth the effort.

*SHOULDERSTAND VARIATIONS (SARVANGASANA)

I. *Benefits:*

The Shoulderstand. . .
- is a cure-all for most *common ailments.*
- improves the *circulation* to such important areas as the *brain,* the *spine,* the *pelvic area;* these are areas which, due to an upright position, rarely receive a good supply of rich, newly-oxygenated blood.
- presses the chin against the thyroid gland which stimulates it and *reduces excess fat.*
- tones up the central *nervous system* and soothes it (tension, insomnia) and is a marvellous rejuvenator.
- has a beneficial effect on the *hormone-producing glands* of the body.
- relieves *palpitation, breathlessness, bronchitis, throat ailments* and *asthma* due to increased circulation to neck and chest.
- relieves pressure on abdominal organs due to body-inversion, which, in turn, regulates the *digestive processes,* frees the body of toxins and increases the *energy-level.*
- is beneficial for *urinary disorders, menstrual troubles* and *piles.*
- relieves *varicose veins* and *aching legs.*
- gives new vitality to people who suffer from *anemia* or *lack of energy.*
- relaxes *whole body.*
- rejuvenates the *sexual glands* and *organs.*
- stretches the *spine.*
- strengthens and firms the muscles of the *back, legs, neck* and *abdomen.*

II. *Technique:*

Variation 1:
1. Lie on the floor, legs out-stretched, hands close by your side, palms down.
2. EXHALE and slowly lift your legs by tensing the abdominal and leg muscles, until they are perpendicular to the floor.
3. Press down on your hands, making them hollow or tent-like. Take 2 breaths.
4. EXHALE, raise your buttocks and lower back and grasp yourself around the waist, with the thumbs around the front of the body. DO NOT let the elbows flare out. This constitutes a Half Shoulderstand.
5. Straighten the legs and tuck the bottom in as much as balance permits.
6. If you are balancing well, then grasp yourself up higher on the rib-cage and tuck your bottom in. (Figure 115)
7. Stretch your legs and point your toes. Hold the position from 10-60 seconds, as a beginner. Gradually work up to 3 minutes. Breathe normally throughout.

*Basic pose described in ABC of Yoga.

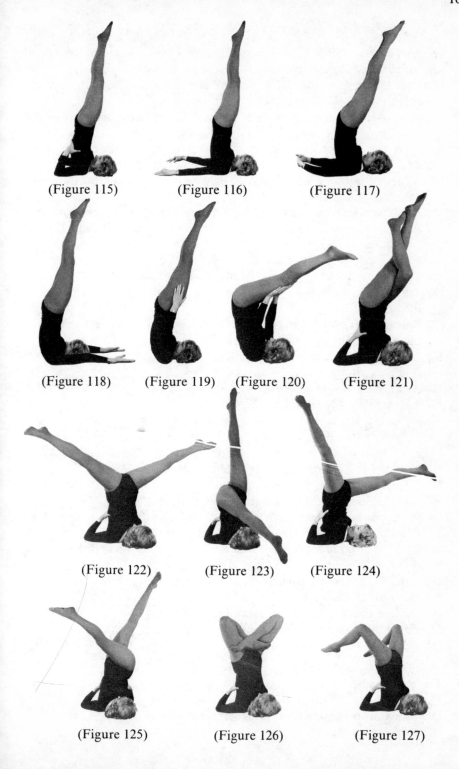

(Figure 115)   (Figure 116)   (Figure 117)

(Figure 118)   (Figure 119)   (Figure 120)   (Figure 121)

(Figure 122)   (Figure 123)   (Figure 124)

(Figure 125)   (Figure 126)   (Figure 127)

Variations-On-A-Theme:

When you are strong enough to be quite straight and confident in SARVANGASANA, you may practice these variations for extra benefits and for variety's sake:

1. Shift the weight to the neck, remove the hands and bring them down behind the back. (Figure 116)
2. As above, clasp the fingers, turn the wrist, so that the thumbs are on the floor, the palms facing away from the body. (Figure 117)
3. Shift the weight, remove the hands, balance and bring the arms stretched out on the floor beside the ears, palms up. (Figure 118)
4. As above, but concentrate on keeping your balance and bring the hands beside the knee. (Figure 119)
5. As above, but place the out-stretched arms against the thighs, and shift the weight to the hands, leaning the body toward the head. (Pose of Tranquility) (Figure 120)
6. Cross your ankles OR assume an Eagle Position. (Figure 121)
7. Spread the legs to the sides. (Figure 122)
8. Spread the legs as you would while walking, one leg pointing forward, the other pointing back. (Figure 123)
9. Spread the legs and then twist from the waist, leaving the legs absolutely immobile in the hip joints. (Figure 124)
10. Cross the thighs and in this position spread them as far as possible. (Figure 125)
11. As above, but with a twist in the waist.
12. Assume the Lotus Position. (Figure 126)
13. Bend the knees and let them hang loosely behind the back, toes pointing to the floor, back arched. (Figure 127)
14. Assume a tripod position, the soles of the feet touching, the knees sideways in a straight line with the body. (Figure 128)
15. Bring one leg straight down on the side, in line with the body, leaving the other up. Repeat on the other side. (Figure 129)
16. Bring one leg straight down in front, the toes on the floor in front of the face. Leave the other leg pointing up. Repeat on the other side.
17 Twist your body to the side, with the legs together, so that the toes are pointing at right angles to the body. (Figure 130)
18. Bend the knees and place them on the forehead. (Figure 131)
19. Go into the Plough Pose.
20. Go into the Bridge Pose. (Figure 132)
21. Point the toes toward each other and push up with the heels, toes pulling down. (Figure 133)

III. *Dos and Don'ts:*

DO tuck your bottom in for a straighter look.
DO stretch your toes up.

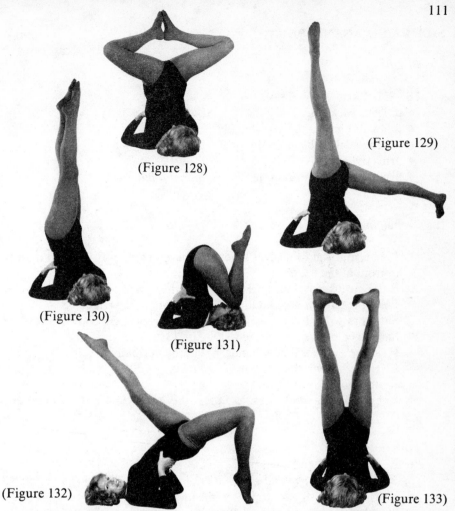

(Figure 128)

(Figure 129)

(Figure 130)

(Figure 131)

(Figure 132)

(Figure 133)

DO NOT get alarmed if you feel slightly dizzy or heady at first. It is quite normal and can be blamed on the sudden dilation of the blood vessels. But do check with your doctor, if you have any doubts. See the basics of Yoga for those who must not practice inverted postures.

DO be patient with yourself. The important thing is to be up there at all, even if it is not a complete shoulderstand for some time.

The Shoulderstand is the second most important pose in Yoga. For many it is the King, since they can not hope to do a Headstand for months or years. Nor is this necessary if this panacea for all ills is practised regularly. The Reverse Shoulderstand (or Half-Shoulderstand, where the hands support the body at the waist) is a most respectable pose in its own right. To do it well and for longer periods, is more important than doing the full Shoulderstand badly. The benefits of the Half-Shoulderstand are especially beneficial to the sex glands.

SIDE RAISE (ANANTASANA)

I. *Benefits:*

The Side Raise...
- relieves *backache.*
- tones and makes the *legs* shapely.
- is beneficial to the entire *pelvic area.*
- firms the *arms.*
- firms and reduces fat in the *thighs, hips* and *buttocks.*

II. *Technique:*

1. Lie on your right side, legs together, the right arm out-stretched slightly in front of the head.
2. Raise the head and support it with your right palm covering half the ear. Place the left hand, palm down, just in front of the chest.
3. Slowly raise the left leg as far as it will go, keeping the body in a straight line. Keep both knees straight. (Figure 134)
4. Hold the pose for 5-20 seconds, breathing normally.
5. EXHALE, lower the leg slowly and relax.
6. Repeat on the other side.
7. Repeat, lifting both legs together, the knees and ankles touching. (Figure 135)

Variation 1:
1. Repeat steps 1 and 2 as above.
3. Bend the right knee and grasp the right toes with the the right hand.
4. EXHALE and slowly straighten the knee.
5. Now bend the elbow and gently pull on the foot, stretching the leg as far up as possible. (Figure 136)
6. EXHALE, lower the leg and relax.
7. Repeat on the other side.

III. *Dos and Don'ts:*

DO have the body in a completely straight line throughout. There is a tendency to stick the bottom out when the leg is raised high.
DO move as slowly in lowering the leg as you did in bringing it up.
DO NOT force beyond a point of comfort.
DO try to grasp the big toe between the thumb and index finger, instead of the whole foot.

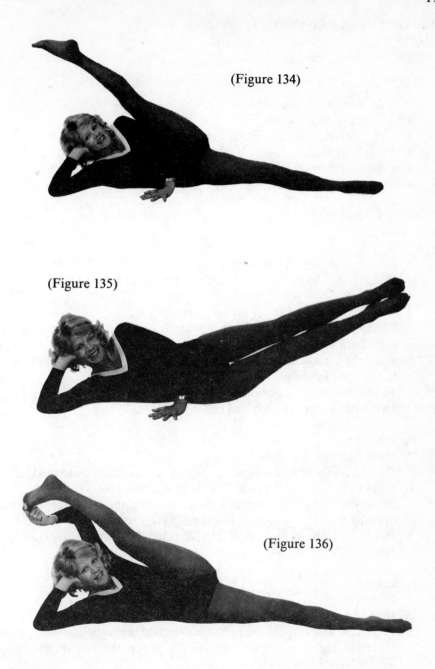

(Figure 134)

(Figure 135)

(Figure 136)

The Side-Raise looks like a calisthenics exercise in slow motion. It is that very slowness that makes for the beautifying and health-restoring results.

SPIDER (SUPTA PADANGUSTHASANA)

I. *Benefits:*

The Spider. . .
- relieves the pain of *sciatica.*
- limbers up the *hip joints.*
- improves *circulation* and tones the *legs.*
- prevents *hernia.*
- is an excellent exercise for people with *paralyzed legs.*
- tightens and firms the *thighs* and *hips.*

II. *Technique:*

1. Lie on your back, the legs extended.
2. Place the left hand on the left leg, bend the right knee and hug it to the chest.
3. Grab the right foot under the toes. (Figure 137)
4. EXHALE, and slowly lift the head, at the same time straightening the right knee and bringing it to the head.
5. Keep the leg straight and pull the leg as much as you can, attempting to touch it with the chin. (Figure 138)
6. Hold for 5-20 seconds, breathing normally.
7. INHALE, lower the body and relax.

Variation 1:
1. Follow steps 1-4 as above.
5. INHALE and bring the right leg slightly forward, and bend the knee.
6. EXHALE, and pull the right foot to the left shoulder.
7. Bring the right elbow up and back, pushing the head through the opening formed by the arm. (Figure 139)
8. Hold for as long as possible. INHALE, bring the bent knee forward and relax.

Variation 2:
1. Follow steps 1-4 as above.
5. INHALE and bring the right leg perpendicular to the floor.
6. EXHALE and keeping the right knee straight throughout, slowly lower the right leg to the floor on the side. Keep the rest of the body motionless. (Figure 140. See page 117.)
7. Hold 5-20 seconds, breathing normally.
8. Release the leg, relax.
9. Repeat all three variations on the other side.

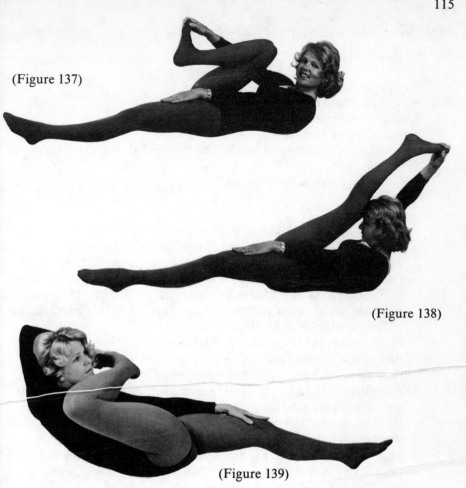

(Figure 137)

(Figure 138)

(Figure 139)

III. *Dos and Don'ts:*

DO keep the outstretched leg absolutely straight and on the floor
throughout.

DO keep the corresponding hand on the outstretched leg.

DO remember it is more important to keep the right leg straight than to
bring the head to the knee.

DO wrap the thumb and index finger around the big toe, if you find it more
effective for you.

The name of the Spider was selected by my children, who thought that that
was what the pose looked like. SUPTA PADANGÜSTHASANA really means:
Lying Down Foot Big Toe Pose. Quite a handle for such a lovely stretching
sensation.

SPONGE

I. *Benefits:*

The Sponge. . .
- promotes deep *muscular relaxation.*
- deeply *relaxes* the *nervous system.*
- restores *peace of mind.*
- results in a reduction of *anxiety* or "nerves" through the release of tension.
- is a marvellous *energy-recharger.*

II. *Technique:*

1. Lie on the floor, legs slightly apart, arms limp by your side.
2. Point your toes away from you and hold for 5 seconds. Relax.
3. Pull the toes up towards the body, bending at the ankle. Hold. Relax.
4. Pull your heels up two inches on the floor and then straighten the legs, pushing the back of the knees firmly against the floor. Hold. Relax.
5. Point the toes toward each other and pull the heels under and up, keeping the legs straight. Hold. Relax.
6. Pinch your buttocks together. Hold. Relax.
7. Pull your abdomen in and up as far as possible. Hold. Relax.
8. Arch the spine back, pushing the chest out. Hold. Relax.
9. With arms straight by your side, palms down, bend the fingers up and back toward the arm, bending at the wrist. Hold. Relax.
10. Bend the elbows and repeat step 9, bending the hands back toward the shoulders. Hold. Relax.
11. Make a tight fist of your hands, bring the arms out to the sides and move the arms up perpendicular to the floor. Move very slowly, resisting the movement all the while to make the pectoral muscles of the bust stand out.
12. Pull the shoulderblades of the back together. Hold. Relax.
13. Pull the shoulders up beside the ears. Hold. Relax.
14. Pull down the corners of the mouth. Hold. Relax.
15. Bring the tongue to the back of the roof of the mouth. Hold. Relax.
16. Purse your lips, wrinkle the nose and squeeze the eyes tightly shut. Hold. Relax.
17. Smile with the lips closed and stretch the face. Hold. Relax.
18. Yawn very slowly, resisting the movement.
19. Press the back of the head against the floor. Hold. Relax.
20. Frown, moving the scalp forward. Hold. Relax.
21. Go through the eye exercises.
22. Pull your head under and against the shoulders without moving anything else.
23. Press the back of your head against the floor. Hold. Relax.
24. Relax, melting into the floor, for up to ten minutes.

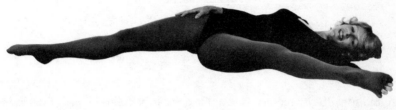

(Figure 140)

III. *Dos and Don'ts:*

DO hold each holding position for at least 5 seconds.

DO relax after each holding position, by flopping back into place after each flexing position.

DO NOT worry or think of unpleasant things as you relax at the end of the Sponge. Rather keep your thoughts to a minimum, on pleasant things, and dispassionately watch them wander past without trying to become involved.

The Sponge is called the Dead Man's Pose or Corpse in the Sanskrit language. Really, it is a deep relaxation pose where your body has a chance to assimilate what it has learned, at its leisure. Seldom do we take the time simply to relax. We may read, watch T.V. or sleep. Just because we lie down does not at all mean we are relaxing our deep-seated neuro-muscular tensions. The body has to relearn how to do that. After some weeks of the deliberate Sponge technique you will find that you can relax without going through all the steps.

*SPREAD LEG STRETCH STANDING (PRASARITA PADOT-TANASANA)

I. *Benefits:*

Standing. . .
- has *weight-reducing* tendencies.
- improves the *circulation* to the *upper body* and *head,* therefore. . .
- gives a feeling of *energy* and *alertness.*
- stretches and develops the *leg muscles* and makes the *legs shapely.*
- is recommended *instead* of the *Headstand* for people with *high blood pressure.*
- is the best forward bend for people with *disc problems.*

II. *Technique:*

1. Stand with the feet as wide apart as possible (4½-5 feet). (Figure 141)
2. Place the hands at the waist, EXHALE, and bend slowly forward from the waist, keeping the back arched back. (Figure 142)
3. When the body is parallel to the floor, bring the hands down in line with the feet, fingers pointing forward.
4. INHALE and bring the head up.
5. EXHALE and lower the crown of the head to the floor in line with the hands, by bending the elbows. (Figure 143)
6. Hold the pose for 10-30 seconds, breathing deeply.
7. EXHALE, straighten up and relax. Repeat if necessary.

III. *Dos and Don'ts:*

DO keep the knees absolutely straight by tightening the knee caps.
DO have the feet, the hands and the crown of the head all in a line.
DO NOT bend the back forward but keep a concave curve.

*Basic Pose described in ABC of Yoga.

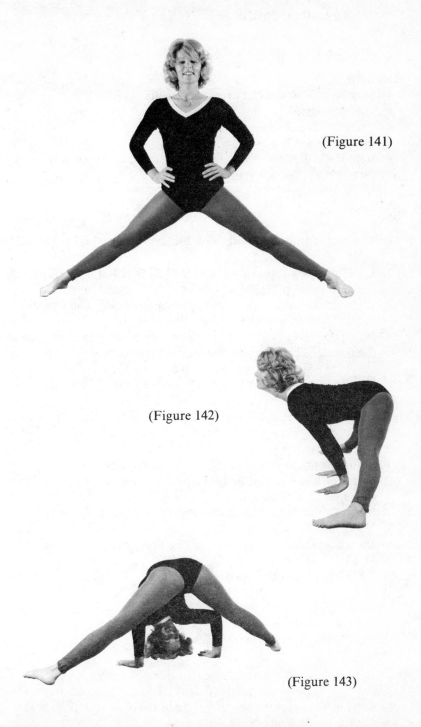

(Figure 141)

(Figure 142)

(Figure 143)

STAFF (DANDASANA, PARIPURNA NAVASANA)

I. *Benefits:*

The Staff. . .
- reduces and removes *fat* from the waistline.
- relieves *stomach gas* and *gastric troubles.*
- is beneficial to the *kidneys.*
- promotes *poise* and *grace.*
- strengthens the *lower back* (for childbearing, elderly people, etc.)
- Variation 1 relieves severe *backache.*

II. *Technique:*

1. Sit on your tailbone on the floor, the legs outstretched, the hands by the hips.
2. EXHALE, bend the elbows, lean slightly backward and slowly raise the legs, the knees straight.
3. Concentrate fiercely, as in any balancing exercise, and attempt to bring the feet on a level with the head. (Figure 144)
4. When you have established balance, slowly bring the hands parallel to the floor, the palms facing the legs. (Figure 145)
5. Hold the pose for as long as you can, or 10-30 seconds.
6. The breathing rhythm should be one of INHALE, EXHALE, hold a little, INHALE, etc. . .
7. EXHALE, lower the legs and relax.

Variation 1:
1. Sit on the floor on your tailbone, the legs outstretched.
2. Bend the knees, bring the heels close to the body and grasp the toes by digging under them with the fingertips.
3. Slowly lift the feet a few inches and establish your balance.
4. EXHALE, concentrate fiercely and slowly straighten the knees stretching the feet onto a level above the head. (Figure 146)
5. Hold, breathing normally, for as long as balance permits.
6. EXHALE, lower the legs and relax.

Variation 2:
1. Follow steps 1-4 as above.
5. Now slowly spread the legs as far as they will go. (Figure 147)

The Staff is an exercise that has specific benefits for all age groups of both sexes. With the proper breathing it works equally well on the abdominal muscles and on the organs, while it strengthens the back as well. In time you will be able to whip into it in one fluid motion.

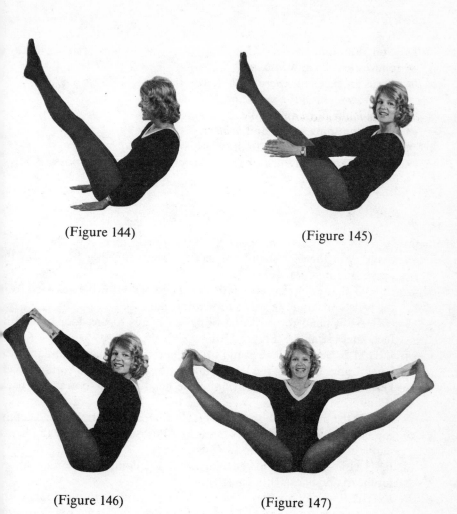

(Figure 144)

(Figure 145)

(Figure 146)

(Figure 147)

I. *Dos and Don'ts:*

DO establish your point of balance by just lifting the feet an inch or two before going into the exercise proper.

DO hold onto the legs near the knees at first for extra support.

DO concentrate on your balance—staring at one spot helps.

DO NOT get discouraged if you keep rolling over on your back. Just practice the Tree and other such balancing exercises, and the back strengtheners listed in the back of the book.

SUN SALUTATIONS (SURYA NAMASKAR)

I. *Benefits:*

The Sun Salutations Pose. . .
- relieves *tension* and *insomnia.*
- acts as an excellent *energizer* and *warm-up.*
- reduces weight in the *waist* and *abdomen.*
- expands the *chest* and makes *breathing easier.*
- makes the spine *supple* and *healthy.*
- improves the *circulation* to the whole body.
- prepares and *strengthens* the *muscles* for more advanced poses.
- increases *stamina.*

II. *Technique:*

1. Stand with the feet slightly apart, the hands together in front of the chest. (Figure 148)
2. INHALE, raise the arms over the head and bend slowly backward from the waist, pushing the pelvis forward. (Figure 149)
3. EXHALE, bend forward and bring the hands to the floor beside the feet, knees straight. (Figure 150)
4. INHALE, bend the knees and bring the right foot back (similar to the Deep Lunge), resting the left thigh on the calf. Keep the bottom down keep the right knee straight, raise the head and try to arch the back (Figure 151)
5. HOLD the breath and bring the left leg alongside the right one, keeping the body in a straight line (similar to a Push-up), with only the hand and toes supporting the body. (Figure 152)
6. EXHALE and slowly lower the body to the floor in this order: knees forehead and chest. (Figure 153)
7. INHALE and in a smooth motion lower the pelvis to the floor, at the same time raising the head and arching the back in a Cobra position (Figure 154)
8. EXHALE, push down on the hands, stick the bottom up, straightening the knees, (similar to a Dog Stretch) and push down on the heels (Figure 155)
9. INHALE and bring the right foot forward setting it down between the hands. Keep the left leg extended, raise the head and arch the back (Figure 156)
10. EXHALE, bring the left leg forward, straighten the knees and perform a Forward Bend, the head as close to the knees as possible. (Figure 157)

11. INHALE, straighten up with the arms over the head and bend back again as far as you can go. (Figure 158)
12. EXHALE, come forward, lower the arms and relax. (Figure 148)
13. Repeat this cycle once more in smooth, fluid motions, eventually working up to 12 repetitions.

III. *Dos and Don'ts:*

DO "PAUSE" for just a moment, rather than "HOLD" at the limit of each position.

DO think of your movements as rhythmic forward and back undulations of the spine. Enjoy the alternating stretches.

DO concentrate on the proper breathing technique.

DO each position to the best of your ability but without undue strain.

DO straighten the outstretched leg in steps 4 and 9, but keep the knees and the tucked-under toes touching the floor.

DO raise the head and arch the back in steps 4 and 9. This means that the bottom is tucked in.

The Sun Salutations are ritually performed at dawn and are repeated 12 times. The Sun is considered the symbol and source of glowing good health and it will enhance your performance to think of yourself basked in sunlight no matter what the weather is outside your window. Slow, unbroken movements with a constant awareness of the spine makes this a delicious all-round exercise.

124

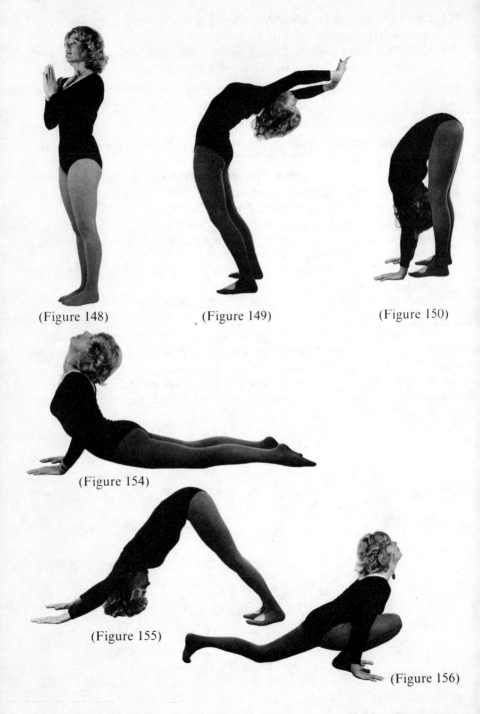

(Figure 148)

(Figure 149)

(Figure 150)

(Figure 154)

(Figure 155)

(Figure 156)

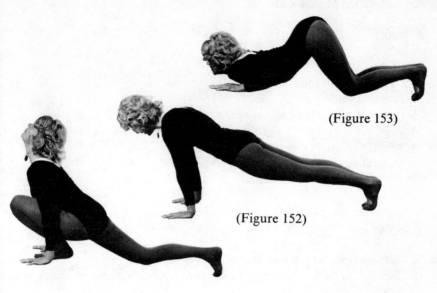

(Figure 153)

(Figure 152)

(Figure 151)

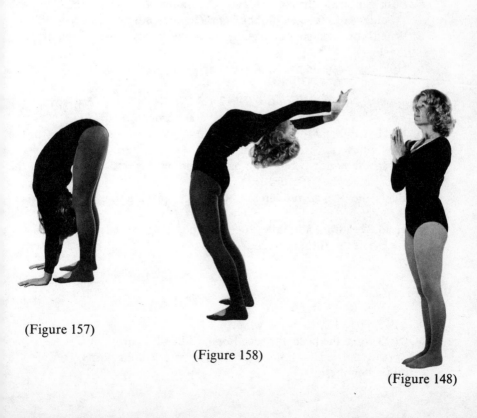

(Figure 157)

(Figure 158)

(Figure 148)

TORTOISE (KURMASANA)

I. *Benefits:*

The Tortoise . . .
- stimulates and tones the *abdominal organs.*
- stretches and tones the *spine.*
- has a calming effect on the *nerves.*
- stretches most muscles of the body, which has a *relaxing effect.*
- gives a feeling of *energy.*
- stimulates the *glands* and *kidneys.*
- stretches and tones the *legs.*

II. *Technique:*

1. Sit on the floor, the legs about 2 feet apart.
2. Bend the knees up slightly, pulling the heels a few inches closer to the body.
3. EXHALE, bend forward and slide the right arm under the bent right knee, then the left arm under the left knee.
4. Push the arms through sideways as much as possible, bringing the shoulders and the head to the floor. (Figure 160)
5. When you can go no further, push the knees down, straightening the legs.
6. Hold this position for 10-60 seconds, *breathing normally.*

Variation 1: Sleeping Tortoise (SVATA KURMASANA) (Very Advanced)
1. Follow steps 1-4 as above. Take several normal breaths.
5. EXHALE, bend the knees slightly and slide the arms back towards the hips, elbows straight, palms up.
6. Clasp the hands behind the back, bending the elbows and lifting the chest somewhat. (Figure 161)
7. Bend the knees and cross the ankles, placing the head between the feet.
8. Hold, breathing normally, 10-20 seconds. (Figure 162)
9. EXHALE, unfurl and relax.

III. *Dos and Don'ts:*

DO NOT spread the legs too wide.
DO NOT force the pose. Practice Forward Bends instead.
DO spread the legs a little after having inserted the arms, in order to straighten them.

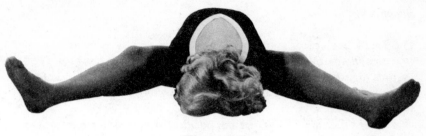

(Figure 160)

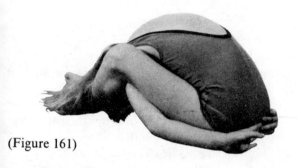

(Figure 161)

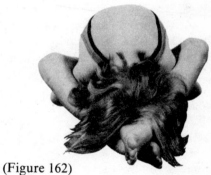

(Figure 162)

DO stretch the arms and neck forward for a perfect pose.

DO attempt to bring the chest and the front of the face to the floor eventually.

DO stretch the arms enough so that they are positioned under the armpits.

The Tortoise is a very advanced pose and should be treated with respect. In its variations it is sacred since it signifies sense withdrawal, meditation.

TRUNK SEALER (MAHA MUDRA)

I. *Benefits:*

The Trunk Sealer . . .
- cures *indigestion.*
- aids *digestion* even with foods that normally can cause discomfort.
- massages and stimulates all *abdominal organs.*
- tones the *kidneys.*
- restores the *womb* to its original position after childbirth or prolapse.
- is of benefit to a man with an enlarged *prostate gland.*
- relieves *hemorrhoids* (piles).

II. *Technique:*

1. Sit on the floor, the legs outstretched, about a foot apart.
2. Bend the left knee, bringing the heel to the groin, the sole of the foot against the right thigh.
3. EXHALE, bend forward and grasp the right big toe with both hands.
4. Let the head hang forward, digging the chin into the jugular notch. Stretch the back up, the shoulders slightly rounded.
5. INHALE and pull the abdomen sharply in and up as in the Abdominal Lift. (Figure 163)
6. EXHALE, banging the tummy out.
7. INHALE again, tighten the abdomen, hold your breath and then EXHALE. Repeat this cycle for as long as you can, or up to 2 minutes, keeping abdomen tightened.
8. Let the tummy relax, EXHALE and take a rest.

III. *Dos and Don'ts:*

DO practice the Abdominal Lift first to get into the habit of tightening the tummy.

DO assume a position similar to the Alternate Leg Stretch, with the right leg stretched straight ahead, the left knee forming a right angle with it.

DO NOT bring the head to the knee, but press it to the chest.

DO keep the spine stretched up.

DO keep the right leg straight and do not roll onto the side of it.

DO tighten your toes while in the pose.

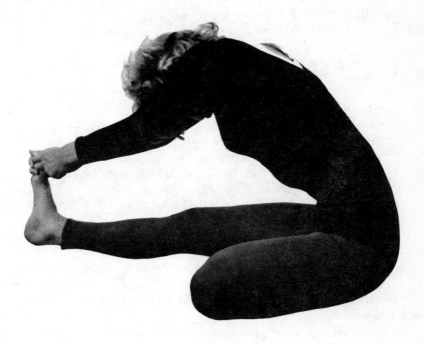

(Figure 163)

The Trunk Sealer is a MUST for abdominal health and is especially good for the man with the paunch, the woman with the Kangaroo pouch. Make it a daily thing between this asana and you.

*TWIST VARIATIONS (ARDHA MATSYENDRASANA)

I. *Benefits:*

The Twist . . .
- firms and reduces *waist.*
- makes the *hipjoint* flexible.
- massages *abdominal organs* to aid digestion.
- makes *spine* limber which has therapeutic effect on the *nervous system.*
- realigns *vertebrae* and relieves *tension.*
- tones *muscles* and *firms figure.*

II. *Technique:*

Variation 1:
1. Sit on the floor, legs outstretched.
2. Spread your legs and bring the *right foot* against the *left thigh.* Press the side of the right knee against the floor.
3. Bend your left knee and, leaving it sticking up in the air, bring the *left foot* over the *right knee.*
4. Set the sole of the *left foot* squarely on the floor. The further back you can bring the foot, the better.
5. Using both hands for support, shift your weight well forward onto the pelvis, to prevent tipping.
6. With the *left hand* behind you on the floor for support, raise your *right arm* and bring it between your chest and the left knee. (Figure 164)
7. Twist your body so that your *right shoulder* is resting against the *left knee.*
8. Now make a fist of your *right hand* and move your *right arm* poker-straight over the *right knee* that is lying on the floor.
9. Attempt to get hold of the toes of the left foot. As a beginner, that is nearly impossible, so it is perfectly all right to grasp the right knee.
10. Levering yourself against the *left leg* with the *right arm,* now twist to the left.
11. Bend your left arm and bring the back of the hand against the small of the back. (Figure 165)
12. Turn your head to the left and look as far left as you can.
13. Hold this position for 10-30 seconds.
14. Slowly unwind.
15. Repeat on the other side.

*Basic pose is described in ABC of Yoga

Variation 2:

For a toning up of the nervous system and a strong, supple back.

1. Follow steps 1-4 bringing the left heel back as close to the hip as possible.
5. Continue with steps 5-8 as above.
9. Now get a good hold of the right knee.
10. EXHALE, and twist the body to the left, swinging the left arm from the shoulder, and bring it around the back. (Figure 166)
11. Grasp the left ankle. Hold 10-30 seconds. Repeat on the other side. (Figure 167)

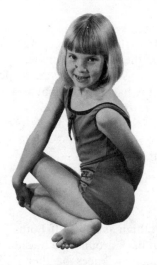

(Figure 164)

Petra Zebroff Age 6

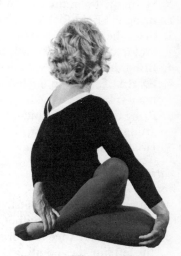

(Figure 165)

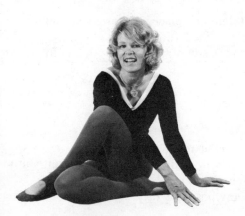

(Figure 166)

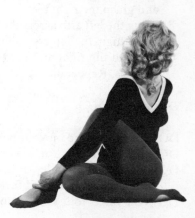

(Figure 167)

Variation 3

For a good abdominal massage, better digestion and elimination of toxins.

1. Sit on the floor, legs outstretched.
2. Spread your legs and bring the right foot to the left thigh. Clasp the foot with both hands and gently lift it as high up and as close to the groin as possible.
3. Proceed as in the original Twist (steps 3-15).

Variation 4:

For backaches, lumbago, hip pains and displaced shoulders.

1. Sit on the floor, the legs outstretched.
2. Bring the right foot against the left thigh.
3. Place the hands beside the hips and lift up the buttocks, sliding the right foot under them. You will be sitting on the side of the ankle.
4. Bring the left foot over the right knee, the sole squarely on the floor.
5. EXHALE, twist to the left and bring the back of the right arm around the left knee bending the elbow. (Figure 168)
6. Bring the left arm around the back and clasp the two hands, preferably around the other wrist.
7. Hold 10-30 seconds. Repeat on the other side.

Variation 5:

For the Arthritic.

1. Sit on the floor, legs outstretched.
2. Gently place the right foot on the left thigh as in a Half-Lotus.
3. Bend the left knee and bring the foot back around the outside against the left hip, toes pointing sideways. Keep the knees together as much as possible.
4. EXHALE, turn to the right, and bring the right arm around the back and grasp the right toes.
5. Bring the left arm across the thighs and place it, elbow locked under the right thigh, the fingers pointing to the left.
6. Twist to the right and hold the position and the foot tightly for 10-30 seconds. Repeat on the other side.

III. *Dos and Don'ts:*

DO sit well forward on your pelvis.
DO NOT bend your arm as you draw it across the knee.
DO swivel your shoulder or upper arm against the knee to permit you to bring your arm around further.
DO NOT force your knees into any positions they do not want to assume easily.
DO exhale and twist as far as you can before you use your arm as leverage. Take a couple of breaths, then exercise and twist as you should.

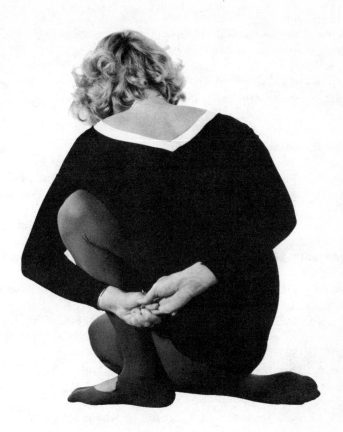

(Figure 168)

The Twist seems like an almost impossible position to assume at first. A picture here is worth 1,000 words. Once you have the idea, however, the Twist will become a most satisfying exercise because it stretches most muscles of the body. A spiral twist to the spine also provides a vigorous abdominal massage, a toning of the kidneys, it increases circulation to the abdominal area and has a calming influence on the shoulders, back and hips of the arthritic. Keep twisting.

WHEEL (URDHVA DHANURASANA OR CHAKRASANA)

I. *Benefits:*

The Wheel . . .
- stretches the *spine* completely and makes the body *supple.*
- is a great *energizer.*
- has a *flattening* effect on the *abdomen.*
- firms the *thighs*
- expands the *chest* for easier *breathing.*
- develops the pectoral muscles of the *bustline.*
- has a tightening effect on the *buttocks.*
- strengthens *arms* and *wrists.*
- improves *circulation* to the *head* and has a soothing effect.
- Variation 1 exercises and strengthens the *feet, ankles* and *knees.*

II. *Technique:*

1. Lie on your back, legs outstretched, arms by your side.
2. Bend both knees and bring the heels as close to the buttocks as possible.
3. Grab the ankles with the hands and pull the heels even closer, keeping them about 1½ feet (a pelvic's width) apart.
4. Bring the hands forward, up and over, placing them on the floor beside the head, a shoulder's width apart, THE FINGERS POINTING TOWARDS THE SHOULDERS. (Figure 169)
5. EXHALE, push down on the hands and raise the body, resting the crown of the head on the floor. Take a few normal breaths. (Figure 170)
6. EXHALE and arch the back, lifting the whole body and shifting the weight to the hands and feet.
7. Stretch the hips up and straighten the arms and legs as much as possible.
8. Hold, breathing normally, from 10-60 seconds.
9. EXHALE, slowly lower the body and relax.

Variations-on a Theme 1:
1. Follow steps 1-7 as above.
8. Now shift your body weight onto the left leg and slowly raise the right leg, parallel to the floor. Hold the position for 10-30 seconds. Repeat on the other side. (Figure 171)

Variations-on-a-Theme 2:
As above, but now raise the right arm as well and place it on the right thigh. Hold for as long as you can. Return the arm and leg to the floor, lower the body and relax. Repeat on the other side.

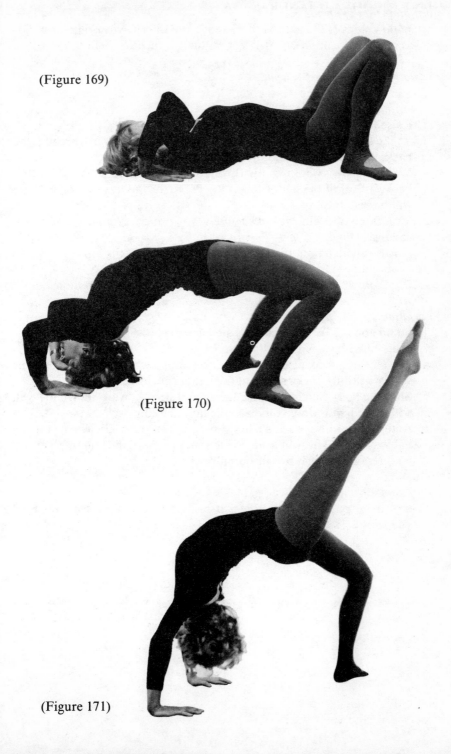

(Figure 169)

(Figure 170)

(Figure 171)

Variations-on-a-Theme 3:
Follow steps 1-7 as in the Wheel above and then slowly bring the hands as close to the heels as possible, eventually touching them.

Variation 1 - Advanced Wheel:
1. Stand straight, the feet about a foot and a half apart, arms by your side.
2. Raise the arms over the head, palms up.
3. At the same time, EXHALE and push the pelvis forward, arching the back. Bend the knees and the back slightly.
4. With the eyes looking up throughout, continue slowly bending backward until the hands touch the floor (for the last foot or so there will be fast drop).
5. Straighten the elbows *immediately* you touch ground or you will collapse. (Figure 172)
6. Now straighten both the arms and legs and stretch the hips up.
7. Hold the pose from 10-60 seconds. Lower the body, relax.
8. For those who find this pose too advanced at first, do Variation 2.

Variation 2:
1. Stand about 3 feet from a wall, the back towards it.
2. Proceed with steps 1-3 in Variation 1.
4. With the eyes looking up in their sockets and back throughout, continue slowly bending backward until the hands touch the wall.
5. Shift the body weight onto the thighs and slowly "walk" down the wall with your hands until you reach the floor. Hold.
6. Return the same way, pushing away from the wall when you are halfway back. This will train you to stand up from the floor in a reverse manner of coming down in Variation 3.

Variation 3:
(Very Advanced). Perform a Wheel by bringing the legs to the floor behind you from a Handstand. (Figure 173)

The Wheel is, like the Lotus, an "either or" posture. Some people, especially children, are able to do it immediately, others need to work hard. As a front-stretching and spine conditioning asana, the wheel cannot be surpassed.

III. *Dos and Don'ts:*

DO come up on your toes after step 7 of the original Wheel. This will give an extra good arch to the spine. Then, without collapsing the arch, slowly lower the heels to the floor.

DO place a small pillow on the floor behind your heels to give you confidence.

DO keep your head completely bent back, the eyes looking up in their sockets.

DO tighten the thighs for a good arch.

DO NOT come up on your toes during step 5.

DO concentrate on getting a good arch in the back, rather than bending the knees, on your downward journey in Variation 3. This is of utmost importance.

DO straighten the elbows immediately on contact with the floor in Variation 1. The motion can be compared to the action of springs in a car. There is a slight give, then the straightening.

DO use a friend for support the first few times you practice Variation 1.

DO NOT attempt any pose that is beyond your ability without strengtheningTHE MUSCLES INVOLVED first.

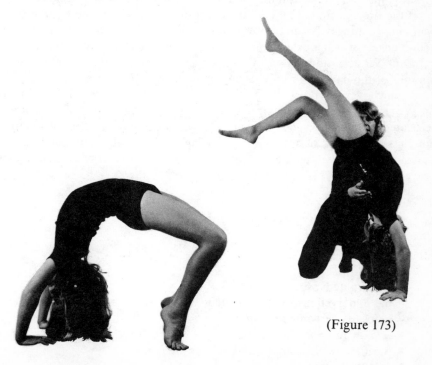

(Figure 173)

(Figure 172)

BREATHING EXERCISES

Considering that we can only live four minutes or so without oxygen, whereas food can be dispensed with for months, we pay very little attention to this great source of energy. Oxygen influences our emotions, helps us to digest our food, repairs cell damage and rids the body of waste matter. Most people use only one-fifth of their potential lung power because of shallow breathing. Your lungs contract and expand like a bellows up to twenty times a minute. The muscle controlling this action is the diaphragm. It is dome-shaped and inflates the lungs by flattening out, thereby pulling on the intercostal muscles. These, in turn, pull apart the rib-cage and the air is now permitted to flood into the bottom of the pear-shaped lungs. To make the diaphragm flatten out, one must push the abdomen out, which is exactly the opposite of what most of us do when inhaling.

In our Western adaptation of Yoga it is sufficient to deep-breathe for ten minutes of the day, preferably in the open. All breathing is done through the nose, which warms, moistens and cleans the air of impurities. Also, it is there, the Yogis believe, that the prana, or energy, we derive from breathing is separated from the oxygen. If basic rules of an upright carriage, of relatively noiseless breathing, of the abdomen being pushed out when inhaling, and pulled in when exhaling, are observed, the rewards are energy, tranquility and peace of mind.

A. *ALTERNATE NOSTRIL BREATH*

I. Benefits:

The Alternate Nostril Breath. . .
- has a marvellously calming effect on the *nervous system.*
- helps to overcome *insomnia.*
- *relaxes* and *refreshes* the body.
- purifies the *bloodstream* and aerates the *lungs.*
- soothes *headaches.*
- improves *digestion* and *appetite.*
- helps to free the mind of *anxiety* and *depression.*

II. *Technique:*

1. Sit in a comfortably cross-legged position, back straight.
2. Raise your RIGHT hand and place your ringfinger against your LEFT nostril, closing it off.
3. Inhale deeply and slowly through the RIGHT nostril to the count of four.
4. Close off the RIGHT nostril with your thumb and retain the breath for a count of 1-4 seconds.
5. Open the LEFT nostril and exhale to the count of 4-8 seconds. The longer you can make the exhalation, the better. Concentrate on completely emptying the lungs.
6. Breathe in through the same LEFT nostril to the count of 4.
7. Close off the nostril with the ringfinger again and hold to the count of 1-4 seconds.
8. Exhale through the RIGHT nostril to the count of 4-8 seconds. This makes up one round.
9. Repeat these rounds of alternate nostril breathing five more times, or up to ten minutes if you are concerned about insomnia.
10. Practice a ratio of 4:4:8, if at all possible. Increase this to 8:4:8 eventually, then 8:8:8, after some months.

III. *Dos and Don'ts*

DO NOT push yourself with the holding position or by increasing the ratio until you are comfortable doing so.
DO make the breathing rhythmic, smooth and slow. You can work on making it inaudible eventually.
DO practice the Alternate Nostril Breath whenever you need calming—if you are nervous, upset or irritable.

I cannot over-emphasize the importance of this particular breath. The body and mind are closely inter-related and one influences the other to a much greater extent than medicine admitted to for many years. As an all-round "soother" the Alternate Nostril Breath is incomparable.

B. *THE CLEANSING BREATH*
I. *Benefits:*

The Cleansing Breath...
- clears *lungs, sinuses* and nasal passages.
- relieves *colds.*
- tones the *nervous system.*
- strengthens the *lungs, thorax* and *abdomen.*
- purifies the *bloodstream* and clears the *head.*
- aids *digestion.*
- stimulates the *liver, spleen* and *pancreas.*

140

II. *Technique:*

1. Sit in a comfortably cross-legged position or a chair, back straight.
2. Inhale deeply, pushing the abdomen out, and taking in as much air as possible in the space of 1 second. (Figure 130)
3. Whack your abdomen in forcefully to expel the air through the nostrils. The sensation should be one of having been punched in the stomach. (Figure 131)
4. Inhale again by pushing the abdomen out and letting the air rush back into the vacuum created by the exhalation.
5. The whole process, inhalation and exhalation, should take not much more than 1½ seconds. Both should be forceful and will be quite audible.
6. Repeat ten times, follow with a complete breath and repeat ten times more.

III. *Dos and Don'ts:*

DO push the abdomen out as far as you can as you inhale.
DO NOT exhale consciously, but let the action of the abdomen do it for you.

The Cleansing Breath is a cross between the Bellows Breath which is more difficult and the Dynamic Cleansing Breath. It has a marvellous effect of clearing the cobwebs out of your mind and is recommended before any task in which you need energy and mental alertness.

C. *COMPLETE BREATH*

I. *Benefits:*

The Complete Breath. . .
- recharges *energy.*
- purifies the *bloodstream* and enriches it.
- develops *chest* and *diaphragm.*
- strengthens *lungs, thorax* and *abdomen.*
- increases resistance to *colds.*
- calms the *nervous system.*
- aids *digestion.*
- clears up *phlegm.*
- helps to lift *depression.*

II. *Technique:*

1. Sit in a comfortably cross-legged position or in a chair.
2. Straighten your back, which will straighten your thorax for easier breathing.
3. Inhale *slowly* through the nose, breathing deeply, consciously.
4. Take five seconds to fill the lower part of the lungs, by expanding the ribs and pushing the abdomen out.
5. Concentrate on filling the top of the lungs for the next five seconds. This will expand the chest and tighten the abdomen slightly.
6. Hold the breath for 1-5 seconds.
7. Exhale slowly until you have emptied the lungs.
8. Repeat 4-5 times more.

III. *Dos and Don'ts:*

DO establish a rhythmic rise and fall of your abdomen, to promote regular breathing.

DO attempt to breathe inaudibly after you have gotten the knack of deep breathing.

DO NOT slump. For maximum efficiency the thorax must be straight.

DO concentrate on your breathing alone, with your eyes closed, if you wish. It serves to do the technique better but it is also a preparation for meditation.

DO push your abdomen out as you breathe in and pull the abdomen in as you breathe out.

DO give an extra snort as you exhale to rid yourself of stale waste-matter in the bottom of the lungs.

Oxygen is our most important food and the customary shallow breathing of most people can be compared to the hasty swallowing of food: both cause immeasurable health-problems. If you regularly breathe deeply you can revitalize yourself and rid yourself of the chronic fatigue so common to housewives; you can improve your mental outlook, your digestion and your general health by resisting repiratory ailments.

D. *DIGESTIVE CYCLE*

For better digestion.
1. Sit, comfortably cross-legged, hands on knees.
2. Now describe a circle with your upper body in a clockwise movement, by
3. Leaning back exhaling, pulling the abdomen IN, then
4. Bending forward inhaling, pushing the abdomen OUT.
5. Repeat 4 times, then perform the same movement in an anti-clockwise direction. The rhythm is: bend forward—inhale—push tummy OUT; lean backward—exhale—pull tummy IN.

This is an easy, effective abdominal churning for the beginner and with the proper breathing, serves as a breath as well. Do not practice with full stomach, while menstruating, pregnant or while suffering from ulcers.

E. *THE HUMMING BREATH*

For Insomnia.
1. Perform a Complete Breath.
2. The second time, make a soft humming sound while exhaling.
3. Repeat 3-10 times, sounding like a persistent bee.
4. Follow up with the SPONGE.
5. Practice at bedtime in bed, if you have trouble falling asleep.

F. *THE LEGS-UP BREATH*

For Respiratory Problems.
1. Lie on your back, buttocks against a wall, legs up. Cross the ankles, if you like.
2. Keep the arms on the floor but place them above the head, palms up, elbows straight.
3. Perform the Complete Breath three times, increasing the number to ten gradually.
4. *For tired feet*. . . lie as above and visualize immersing your feet into a red hot river when inhaling, then plunging them into a cool green lake when exhaling.
5. *For sinus troubles*. . . lie cross-wise on your bed, face up, head hanging over the edge. Breathe deeply, closing off one nostril while you breathe in and out several times. Repeat with the other nostril, then breathe normally again.

G. RHYTHMIC BREATH

Benefits:
- calms the mind (depression, anxiety)
- gives energy

For a happier you.
1. Sit comfortably cross-legged, spine straight.
2. Place your middle fingers on the wrist, or on the temple to find the pulse.
3. Count to the rhythm of 1, 2, 3; 1, 2, 3, 4, or 1, 2, 3, 4, 5, etc., depending on how long you can hold your breath.
4. When you have committed the rhythm of the pulse to memory, remove your fingers, and start a Complete Breath to the pulse rhythm of IN−1, 2, 3, 4, Hold−1, 2, OUT−1, 2, 3, 4. The Rhythmic Breath has the purpose of bringing you in tune with the universe and therefore rids you of all negative, lonely emotions.
5. Repeat 3-4 times as a beginner, then rest.
6. As you become proficient, increase the breaths by one extra a week until you have worked up to 10 minutes, gradually.

H. WALKING BREATH

This breath falls into the same category as the Rhythmic Breath and it is an excellent way of utilizing fresh air. When you walk to the store, take the dog out, jog, go for a bike-ride, climb steps or walk on the spot, simply suit the rhythm of breath to the steps you take:
IN−1, 2, 3, 4 (or 1, 2, 3, 4, 5, 6, etc); HOLD−1, 2; OUT−1, 2, 3, 4 (or 1, 2, 3, 4, 5, 6, etc). Make this a pleasant habit and you will find many rewards such as increased energy, a calm mind, better digestion and resistance to infection.

J. BREATHING-AWAY-PAIN BREATH

1. Lie on your back and breathe deeply and rhythmically.
2. Think positively that you are going to breathe away the pain.
3. Now direct all your life-force, all the energy you derive from every inhalation, to the pain (a headache, toothache, backache, menstrual pain, etc.) and concentrate on breathing it away with every exhalation.
4. It has been found helpful to drink half a glass of cool water first.

I. SENSE-SEALER

Benefits:

The Sense Sealer. . .
- calms the mind.
- teaches concentration.
- offsets depression, tension and anxiety.
- cures insomnia.

Technique:
1. Sit in a comfortable and cross-legged position, spine straight.
2. Raise your arms so that the elbows are at shoulder height and place the hands on either side of the nose.
3. Now close the eyes, look upwards and place the index and middle fingers on the eyelids.
4. The ring fingers now gently push against the nostrils, the opening an oval rather than a round shape. The little fingers rest somewhere below the nostrils.
5. Now place the thumbs against the earholes and apply gentle pressure on ears and eyes.
6. Breathe normally and concentrate on the deep ebb and flow of your breath. Think of nothing else.
7. Perform only 3-4 breaths at first, increasing this by one breath a week until you are doing it for 5-10 minutes.

The Sense Sealer can be considered one of the bridges between Hatha Yoga and Meditation. It is designed to still the mind, to turn the gaze inward—for peace is to be found nowhere else. Normally, our senses keep us chained to darkness as each one tempts us to follow its desires. Spiritual enlightenment can only come when we are desireless. The serious Yoga student would be wise, also, to look into the tremendously powerful visualization breaths and exercises. Here, the prana, or life-force, is capable of performing miracles with your help. You can breathe away tiredness, breathe away pain, recharge your whole body with the energy and joy of healthful, intelligent living. You can cleanse yourself, cool or warm yourself, or tranquilize yourself. Your energy can be pulled from the sun, the air, the water, the earth; and you can direct this energy to any part of your body or to some-one else in order to heal—all through breathing exercise. Such techniques require the teachings of an expert and have no place in this book. But let us make a small beginning with the Breathing-Away-Pain Breath.

SCHEDULES

1. GENERAL INFORMATION

Immediately upon rising:
1. Stretching—luxuriously while still in bed
2. Abdominal Lift—after a glass of water with lemon juice
3. Breathing—for ten minutes in front of open window

Any time during the day:
1. Warm-ups
2. Headstand, Shoulderstand, i.e. inverted poses
3. Neck and Eye Exercises
4. Stretches
5. Balancing Poses
6. Relaxation—Meditation

The suggested order of exercises varies slightly from author to author, but this is an accepted general outline. Please insert an imaginary "Relaxation" after each category if it is needed for your greater enjoyment or for better performance during your Yoga Exercise period. Remember to alternate forward bending poses with backward bending exercises and to give a little variety by having an alternating over-all program, such as the Short Three Day Course. Expand the time of exercising according to your need or time available, but do practice every day, however briefly. How often you repeat a pose depends on how long you have held it. If, however, you are so advanced that you are in a pose for 30-60 seconds, then you are in the enjoyable position of performing everything only once. For both categories of Yogis there is one common rule: breathe normally, do not hold your breath. Use the suggested breathing rhythm to aid you in more expert performance of each pose. Rest between exercises.

2. SHORT THREE DAY COURSE

To the beginner this course looks most awesome, to the advanced student of Yoga it is a most joyful experience. The poses and their sequence are carefully thought out, but the holding time is a guide only. Suit this to your own capacity. Pay close attention to the breathing rhythm and feel the shackles of an enervating day fall from you.

DAY 1:

Headstand	10 min.
Shoulderstand	10 min.
Plough	5 min.
Leg-Over	30 sec.
Staff	1 min.
Inverted Boat	20-30 sec.
Forward Bend Sitting	1 min.
Marichi's Pose	30 sec.
Twist	30 sec.
Mountain	1 min.
Fish	20-30 sec.
Boat	20-30 sec.
Bow	30 sec.
Cobra-on-Toes	20-30 sec.
Dog Stretch	1 min.
Forward Bend Standing	1-2 min.
Sponge	5 min.
Alternate Nostril	
Complete Breath	

DAY 2:

Headstand with Twist	20 sec.
Headstand 1 leg down	15 sec.
Headstand Lotus	20 sec.
Headstand Lotus, hugging chest	30 sec.
Shoulderstand—inverted palms	30 sec.
Shoulderstand—arms extended	30 sec.
Shoulderstand—arms beside legs	30 sec.
Plough—knees down	30 sec.
Shoulderstand—1 leg down side	20 sec.
Shoulderstand—1 leg in front	20 sec.
Shoulderstand—in Lotus	20 sec.
Alternate Leg Stretch	15 sec.
Alternate Leg Stretch in Half Lotus	20 sec.
Feet apart Forward Bend	20 sec.
Marichi's Pose	20 sec.

Backward Bend	20 sec.
Plough—legs spread	20 sec.
Plough both legs to side	20 sec.
Leg-Over	15 sec.
Pump (arms up)	15 sec.
Trunk Sealer	15 sec.
Sponge	15 sec.
Fwd. Bend Sitting	2 min.
Balancing Fwd. Bend	1 min.
Marichi's Pose other arm	30 sec.
Twist	30 sec.
Knee to Thigh Stretch	1 min.
Forward Bend Standing	2 min.
Sponge	8 min.
Complete Alternate Nostril	8 min.

DAY 3:

Triangle Posture	30 sec.
Respectful Chest Expander	30 sec.
Spread Leg Str. Standing	30 sec.
Forward Bend Standing	30 sec.
Forward Bend, toes, hands under	30 sec.
Eagle	15 sec.
Horseman Pose	15 sec.
Cross Beam	15 sec.
Camel	20 sec.
Cobra	20-30 sec.
Sitting Warrior	30-40 sec.
Reclining Warrior	30-40 sec.
Reclining Warrior in Fish pose	30-40 sec.
Lotus	30 sec.
Mountain	30 sec.
Lotus-pushup	30 sec.
Fish	30 sec.
Posture Clasp	15 sec.
Lion	20 sec.
Forward Bend Sitting	3-5 min.

3. EXPECTANT MOTHERS

1. Mountain
2. Complete breath with suspension, relieved by a short gasp now and then

3. Squat
4. Pelvic Rock
5. Knee & Thigh Stretch
6. Hands-to-Wall

7. Spread Leg Stretch Sitting
8. Sitting Warrior
9. Cross Beam
10. Lying Pelvic Rock

Do check with your doctor on the advisability of practicing Yoga during pregnancy. Generally-speaking it is quite safe to exercise for the first three months if there is no history of miscarriage. After that, do not perform poses which put undue pressure on the abdomen or which are inverted. The lying Pelvic Rock is done lying on the back, the heels drawn up towards the buttocks, knees up. Tilt the pelvis by pressing the small of the back against the floor and hold. A more advanced version is to lift the buttocks off the floor altogether. Both versions are helpful for menstrual pain.

4. POST-NATAL EXERCISES

1. Cat-Stretch—Pelvic Rock
2. Mountain Breathing, keeping arms up
3. Plough Variation—both legs to side
4. Spread Leg Stretch

5. Cross Beam
6. Staff with legs apart
7. Leg—Over
8. Lying Side Stretch

It is important to return the uterus to its normal position and to strengthen the transverse back muscles, whose job it is to knit together the spread bones of the pelvis after childbirth. For the first six weeks the program should consist mainly of stretching poses, such as the Cross Beam and the Lying Side Stretch: lie on your back, arms extended along the sides. Without moving the back against the floor reach with your fingertips along one side as though you wanted to touch your toes. Hold. Repeat on the other side.

5. ESPECIALLY FOR MEN

1. Chest Expander
2. Mountain or Cleansing Breath
3. Peacock
4. Push-Up
5. Alternate Leg Stretch

6. Locust
7. Leg-Over
8. Staff
9. Crow-to-side

Because these exercises develop muscles and keep the prostate gland healthy as well, they are "just for him". Of course, in Yoga there are no "his" or "her" exercises per se and all are equally beneficial for both sexes because Yoga works for internal health. However, the Peacock is considered particularly male.

6. YOGA OVER FORTY

1. Rock 'n Rolls—or Cat Stretch
2. Crossed-Knee Bend or Alternate Nostril Breath
3. Arm and Leg Stretch
4. Knees-to-side or Knee Presses
5. Pose of Tranquility
6. Cobra—Pose of a Child
7. Ankle to Toe Exercises such as Squat
8. Plough with Legs Spread
9. Twist

This may look like a complicated-looking program for the elderly, but it is my experience that, once fear of injury has been overcome, the loosening-up progress is astoundingly fast. Start with a simple version at first, holding positions short, and follow common sense in advancing. Age is an accumulation of bad habits, be it eating, poor posture or shallow breathing, and it will take time to eliminate this. Be patient.

7. YOGA FOR CHILDREN

1. "Follow-the-Leader" Warm-up
2. Cooling Breath
3. Shoulder Stand with all its variations
4. Lotus positions: in Shoulderstand, in the Lion, on the tummy hands in cathedral shape in back, Yoga-Mudra, Walking-in-it, etc.
5. Wheel
6. Forward Bend—Rag Doll, Falling Tree
7. Tortoise (sleeping)
8. Fish (in lotus)
9. Crow—(side ways)
10. Plough into Backward Roll
11. Balancing Poses—being a wing-flapping stork, or Rooster
12. Eagle
13. Swan
14. Sponge—Dead Man's Float

The list of stimulating exercises for children is endless and I am sure that you will find some more. Make Yoga a pleasant game—visualization (pretending) is very much a part of it. Alternate holding poses with active ones, i.e. be a hopping rabbit after the Squat. Teach them the Cooling Breath in fun, then apply it when they have a fever (or you have a craving to be subdued). Let them perform the Cobra very, very slowly, then do a more rapid Woodchopper Breath. Practice the Wheel at first against the wall—back to it, half the body height away from it, crawling down backwards to the floor. When you come up, push away from the wall without coming all the way up. Do that from lower and lower down until the whole maneuver can be performed without a wall. Children are basically more flexible than we adults, but often start out quite stiff. They do loosen up very quickly, though. Practice the Backward Roll by doing a Plough, bringing the hands close to the shoulders, *fingertips pointing to the shoulders* and give a little push with equal pressure on *both* hands. Share the pleasure of Yoga with them.

8. EXERCISES FOR SPECIFIC AREAS

Poses in italics are to be found in ABC of Yoga

ABDOMEN:
   Abdominal Lift, Ankle to Forehead Stretch, Arm and Leg Stretch, Both Forward Bends, Bow, Chest Expander, Cock, Crow, Deep Lunge, Dog Stretch, Ear to Knee Pose, Headstand, Locust, Lotus, Peacock, Plough, Push-Up, Scorpion, Sun Salutations, Tortoise, Trunk Sealer.
   Alternate Leg Stretch, Cross Beam, Leg-Over, Mountain, Pump, Rock 'n Rolls, Sit-Up.

ARMS & WRISTS:
   Ankle to Forehead Stretch, Arm and Leg Stretch, Bow, Chest Expander (Var.), Cobra (Var.), Cock, Cow Head Pose, Crow, Inclined Plane, Peacock, Push-up, Shooting Bow, Side Raise.
   Arm Lift, Cat Stretch, Fountain, Posture Clasp.

ANKLES:

Arm and Leg Stretch, Cobra-on-Toes, Deep Lunge, Dog Stretch, Eagle Pose, Forward Bend Standing, Frog, Horse, Inclined Plane, Lotus, Triangle Postures, Wheel.
Ankle Bends, Cross Beam, Knee and Thigh Stretch, Sitting Warrior.

BACK AND SPINE:

Bow, Bridge, Chest Expander Variations, Cobra, Ear to Knee Pose, Forward Bends, Horse, Locust, Lotus, Marichi's Pose, Plough, Scorpion, Staff, Tortoise, Twist, Wheel.
Alternate Leg Stretch, Boat, Camel, Cat Stretch, Cross Beam, Leg-Over, Pendulum, Pump.

BUST AND CHEST:

Arm and Leg Stretch, Bow, Chest Expander, Cobra, Cow Head Pose, Crow, Fish, Forward Bend Standing, Inclined Plane, Plough, Push-up, Sun Salutations, Wheel, Triangle Postures.
Hands to Wall, Pelvic Stretch, Posture Clasp.

BUTTOCKS:

Bow, Bridge, Cobra, Inclined Plane, Locust, Plough, Push-up, Shoulderstand, Side Raise, Wheel.
Alternate Leg Stretch, Pump, Sit-up.

CIRCULATION:

Chest Expander, Cow Head Pose, Deep Lunge, Dog Stretch, Forward-Bend Standing, Headstand, Marichi's Pose, Peacock, Scorpion, Shoulderstand, Spider, Spread Leg Standing, Sun Salutations, Wheel.
Curling Leaf, Mountain, Pendulum, Pump, Symbol of Yoga.

EYES:

Headstand, Shoulderstand.
Eye Exercises, Lion, Neck Rolls.

FACE:

Forward Bend Standing, Plough, Shoulderstand.
Beauty Breath, Lion, Symbol of Yoga.

FEET:

Balancing on Toes, Forward Bend Sitting, Frog, Perfect Posture, Reclining Warrior, Squat.
Japanese Sitting Position, Pelvic Stretch, Toe Twist.

KNEES:

Arm and Leg Stretch, Forward Bend Sitting, Frog, Horse, Lotus, Twist.
Alternate Leg Stretch, Knee and Thigh Stretch, Sitting Warrior, Toe Exercise.

HIPS:

Ankle to Forehead Stretch, Arm and Leg Stretch, Bow, Chest Expander, Ear to Knee Pose, Horse, Inclined Plane, Leg Split, Plough, Shooting Bow, Side Raise, Spider, Triangle Posture, Twist, Locust.
Fountain.

LEGS:

Arm and Leg Stretch, Bow, Chest Expander, Cow Head Pose, Deep Lunge, Dog Stretch, Eagle Pose, Forward Bend Sitting, Frog, Knee to Ear Pose, Leg Split, Perfect Posture, Reclining Warrior, Shooting Bow, Side Raise, Spread Leg Standing, Tortoise.
Alternate Leg Stretch, Curling Leaf, Stork, Toe Twist, Tree.

LUNGS:

Chest Expander to Side, Headstand, Scorpion.

NECK AND CHIN:

Arm and Leg Stretch, Bridge, Chest Expander, Cobra, Crow, Fish, Knee Press, Plough.
Cat Stretch, Neck Rolls.

PELVIC AREA:

Cobra, Ear to Knee Pose, Locust, Reclining Warrior, Side Raise.

POSTURE AND SHOULDERS:

Arm and Leg Stretch, Bow, Chest Expander, Cobra, Cock, Cow Head Pose, Eagle Pose, Forward Bend Standing, Lotus, Plough.
Arm Lift, Blade, Camel, Pelvic Stretch, Pendulum, Posture Clasp, Tree, Stork.

THIGHS:

Ankle to Forehead Stretch, Arm and Leg Stretch, Deep Lunge, Eagle Pose, Forward Bend Standing, Horse, Inclined Plane, Leg Split, Perfect Posture, Reclining Warrior, Shooting Bow Pose, Side Raise, Spider, Spread Leg Stretch, Triangle Posture, Wheel.
Alternate Leg Stretch, Crossed Beam, Knee and Thigh Stretch, Pelvic Stetch.

TOES:

Push-up, Cobra-on-Toes.
Pelvic Stretch, Toe Balance, Toe Twist.

WAIST AND MIDRIFF:

Abdominal Lift, Bridge, Ear to Knee Pose, Sun Salutations, Triangle Posture, Twist.
Fountain, Leg-Over, Pump, Toe Twist.

9. EXERCISES FOR HEALTH PROBLEMS

ANEMIA:
Both Forward Bends, Complete Breath, Shoulderstand, Sponge.

ARTHRITIS:
Cobra, Cow Head Pose, Dog Stretch, Forward Bend Standing, Shoulderstand, Triangle Posture, Locust, Twist.
Curling Leaf, Mountain.

ASTHMA:
Arm and Leg Stretch, Both Forward Bends, Cobra, Fish, Headstand, Locust, Reclining Warrior, Shoulderstand .
Alternate Leg Stretch, Mountain.

BURSITIS:
Chest Expander, Cow Head Pose.
Blade, Pendulum, Posture Clasp.

BACHACHE:
All standing poses, Bow, Cobra, Crossed Knee Bend, Ear to Knee Pose, Forward Bend Sitting, Knee Press, Shoulderstand, Side Raise, Trunk Sealer.
Alternate Leg Stretch, Leg-Over.

BALANCE AND POISE:
Cock, Crow, Deep Lunge, Eagle Pose, Forward Bend Sitting, Leg Split, Scorpion, Staff.

BREATHLESSNESS:
All breathing exercises, Both Forward Bends, Plough, Shoulderstand, Sponge.
Mountain.

COMMON COLD:
Both Forward Bends, Complete Breath, Headstand, Shoulderstand.

CONSTIPATION:
Abdominal Lift, Both Forward Bends, Bow, Chest Expander, Fish, Headstand, Knee Press, Plough, Shooting Bow, Shoulderstand, Squat, Triangle Postures, Twist, Yoga Mudra.
Alternate Leg Stretch, Toe Exercises.

DIABETES:
>Fish, Forward Bend Sitting, Locust, Peacock, Plough, Shoulderstand, Twist, Trunk Sealer.
>*Alternate Leg Stretch, Mountain.*

DIGESTION:
>See Constipation and Indigestion.

DISPLACED DISC:
>All Standing Postures, Bow, Camel, Cobra, Forward Bend Sitting, Locust, Shoulderstand.
>*Cat Stretch.*

FATIGUE:
>Both Forward Bends, Chest Expander, Complete Breath, Headstand, Plough, Sun Salutations, Shoulderstand, Twist.
>*Ankle Bends, Curling Leaf.*

FLAT FEET:
>Frog, Sitting and Reclining Warrior, Shoulderstand.
>*Knee and Thigh Stretch.*

GALL BLADDER:
>Both Forward Bends, Locust, Shoulderstand, Triangle Postures, Twist.
>*Alternate Leg Stretch.*

GLANDS (endocrine, pituitary, pineal):
>Headstand, Tortoise.

HEADACHE:
>Alternate Nostril Breathing Without Retention, Forward Bends, Headstand, Plough, Shoulderstand (for 3 mins. or more).
>*Thigh Exercises, Neck Rolls.*

HEART TROUBLE:
>Complete and Alternate Nostril Without Retention.

HEELS (calcaneal spurs or pain):
>Dog Stretch, Frog, Shoulderstand, Sitting Warrior, Triangle (formed by legs on arms on floor, pressing the heels toward the floor).
>*Knee and Thigh Stretch.*

HERNIA PREVENTION:
>Spider.

HIGH BLOOD PRESSURE:

Alternate Nostril Breathing, Dog Stretch, Forward Bend Sitting, Plough, Spread Leg Standing, Sponge.
Alternate Leg Stretch, Symbol of Yoga.

INDIGESTION:

Ankle to Forehead Stretch, Bow, Cobra, Crossed Knee Bend, Locust, Marichi's Pose, Peacock, Plough, Shoulderstand, Staff, Trunk Sealer.
Mountain, Pump, Symbol of Yoga.

INSOMNIA:

Alternate Nostril Breathing, Bellows Breath, Cobra, Forward Bend Sitting, Headstand, Plough, Shoulderstand, Sun Salutations.
Mountain, Neck Rolls.

KIDNEYS:

Bow, Cobra-On-Toes, Ear to Knee Pose, Forward Bend Sitting, Locust, Plough, Shoulderstand, Spread Leg Stretch, Staff, Standing, Tortoise, Trunk Sealer.
Knee and Thigh Stretch, Leg-Over, Twist.

LUMBAGO:

Bow, Cobra, Locust, Plough, Sponge.

MENSTRUAL DISORDERS AND OVARIES:

Both Forward Bends, Cobra, Dog Stretch (advanced), Fish, Shoulderstand, Sitting and Reclining Warrior, Spread Leg Stretch, Triangle Postures.
Symbol of Yoga, Mountain, Knee and Thigh Stretch, Cat Stretch.

OBESITY AND WEIGHT CONTROL:

Both Forward Bends, Cobra, Fish, Knee Press, Locust, Plough, Shoulderstand, Spread Leg Stretch Standing, Triangle Postures, Twist, Wheel.

PALPITATIONS:

Alternate Nostril Breath Without Retention at the beginning, Both Forward Bends, Complete Breath, Dog Stretch (advanced), Headstand, Plough, Shoulderstand, Sitting Warrior, Sponge.

PILES:

Bow, Fish, Locust (Boat), Plough, Shoulderstand, Trunk Sealer.
Leg-Over.

PROSTATES:

Bow, Dog Stretch (advanced), Forward Bend Standing, Lotus, Sitting and Reclining Warrior.
Leg-Over, Locust (Boat), Staff (advanced), Alternate Leg Stretch.

RHEUMATISM:

Forward Bend Sitting, Plough, Reclining Warrior, Twist, Shoulderstand.
Mountain, Boat, Alternate Leg Stretch.

SCIATICA:

Ankle to Forehead Stretch, Both Forward Bends, Bow, Cobra, Leg Split, Shoulderstand, Spider, Spread Leg Stretch.
Leg-Over, Alternate Leg Stretch, Boat.

SEXUAL DEBILITY:

Abdominal Lift, Headstand, Locust, Reclining Warrior, Shoulderstand, Trunk Sealer.
Symbol of Yoga.

SINUS:

Headstand.

SLIMMING:

Abdominal Lift, Bow, Fish, Plough, Shoulderstand, Twist.
Fountain, Pump.

SLIPPED DISC:

See Displaced Disc.

TENSION:

Arm and Leg Stretch, Chest Expander, Cobra, Cow Head Pose, Dog Stretch, Ear to Knee Pose, Forward Bends (Knee and Thigh), Knee Press, Plough, Shoulderstand, Sun Salutations, Sponge, Twist.
Neck Rolls, Lion, Fish, Rock n' Rolls, Alternate Leg Stretch, Eye Exercises, Curling leaf.

NUTRITION

YOU ARE WHAT YOU EAT

If you were to ask me for my favourite thought-of-the-day, I would unhesitatingly quote the Karmic law which in one form or another has appeared in every religion in the world: "As ye sow, so shall ye reap." This thought decrees that your every action has a reaction, every cause an effect. If you plant an apple seed, by and by you will have an apple tree. When you eat one of its fruits you will receive Vitamins A, B, B_2, calcium, some phosphorus, iron, sugar (carbohydrates) and some fat, all for very few calories. If you eat properly and your body receives all the vitamins and minerals it needs you will be glowingly healthy. If you are truly healthy you will have joyous energy to spare, bounce back from any misfortune and spread cheer all around you. If, however, your body is deficient in one element or another, and its miraculous and delicate clockwork mechanism is thrown out of kilter, you become what amounts to a "cripple." Just because your failing is not so obvious to the casual observer as a limp, it is no less a lack. Perhaps you are a premenstrual-grouch cripple because of a need for calcium; or you are a poor-eyesight cripple because of a vitamin A deficiency. It could well be, of course, that your over-weight disfigurement is due to a lack of oil, protein or iron in your diet, or that your poor sore feet are crying for vitamin E. Magnesium, brewer's yeast, iron, protein—I could go on and on throwing amazing tidbits of nutritional facts at you.

When I first started reading such excellent books on nutrition as Linda Clark's STAY YOUNG LONGER, Catharyn Elwood's FEEL LIKE A MILLION, Adelle Davis' LET'S EAT RIGHT TO KEEP FIT, Gayelord Hauser's and Lelord Kordel's books, and such magazines as *LET'S LIVE, PREVENTION,* and *YOGA AND HEALTH,* it was I who was amazed. It seems as though any atheist must find indisputable evidence of a God in the intricate and wonderful workings of the body. Here too, not only does every action have a reaction, but there is a reaction to the reaction. Everything is interdependent. For instance, the healing qualities of Vitamin A are doubled if Vitamin E is also taken; or lecithin helps vitamin A, D, E, K and fat to be carried and absorbed in the body. Another instance is the marvellous vitamin B-complex which is synergistic. That is, the balance between the B- vitamins (over 20 are known and more are being discovered all the time) is most delicate and if you supply too much of one you cause a deficiency of the other.

It is precisely in some of these vitamins that we North Americans are most deficient. That is not at all surprising when you know that one of the most common sources of the B vitamins are liver, brewer's yeast, molasses, whole-wheat cereals and breads. Just how often do YOU partake of these nutritious foods? You may have liver once every three weeks because you vaguely know that it's good for you—but the kids hate it. My children love it. But this may be because I use Adelle Davis' recipe of liver baked with onions and apples, a bit of sherry, some thyme and bits of bacon.

And whole-wheat breads—what's that? In our super-instant, super-refined society the term "bread" often means a gooey, pallid, dead mass which can be squashed better than the softest toilet-paper. These breads and cakes are made of the purest, whitest flour and sugar which have been highly refined so that the bugs don't eat them. The question now is *why* do the bugs not touch them? Because, of course, they instinctively know that these processed products have no food value! They are nothing but calories. Now, it is all very well to eat calories,—indeed, we need about 2000 to 3500 calories daily to produce the energy needed for our work. However, a calory has no nutritional value of its own; it is a unit of measurement only: "X" number of calories produces "Y" amount of heat. Figuratively speaking, there exist two types of calories and they must never be lumped together or poor health may result. Let us take the avocado (350 calories) on the one hand and a piece of banana cream pie (350 calories) on the other. You will say that you cannot afford to eat either, since they are both fattening. Wrong! How can you *NOT* afford to eat such a marvellous fruit as the avocado which has to its credit approximately seventeen vitamins, fourteen minerals, lots of protein, lots of linoleic acid (unsaturated fatty acid) and the like, while the piece of pie has so little nutrients. The fruit is burnt up by the body, its various nutrients being soaked up like a sponge. The pie, partially because it is sugary, is almost immediately stored as fat wherever the body can quickly stuff it for storage. Such a place is almost certainly the tummy, where the loops of the intestines permit easy storage corners. Or it is in that place where YOU tend to show your weight most—the slipped hip, the bust, the thighs, the paunch. Neither can peanuts be considered fattening because they are an excellent source of protein, linoleic acid and vitamins and minerals. It is only when food is devoid of these elements that they become "fattening". So, change your thinking from today onward and, by all means, indulge in nuts and the like, but consider them as a meal in themselves. If they are added to your general caloric intake by being eaten just before a cocktail party, then of course they become fattening—but no more so than all of the other foods you eat then. Rule of thumb: if it is natural, it is usually nutritious. And that is also the simplest way of defining Yoga nutrition. If it is refined or made from white processed super flour, rice, noodles or hydrogenated oils, it is fattening. A slice of whole-wheat bread enriched with wheat-germ, bran, nutritional yeast, molasses, sunflower seeds, rice polishings, cheese, etc., is not fattening; it is a natural source of good, balanced health. Can you say the same of white bread whose grains have been polished and bleached of these very ingredients—even if it is enriched with synthetic vitamins? Children need bread—it is one of the reasons that our forefathers had the energy to expend great physical effort in their hard daily lives, and that heart attacks were considerably fewer. Another needed food, especially in such famine-stricken countries as Ireland and Europe after the wars, was the hardy potato. A medium-sized potato actually has less caloric content than ½ cup of cottage-cheese; however it must be cooked right, always in its jacket. This is a much-maligned vegetable which is really an excellent source of Vitamin C and some protein.

Protein: what is it?
A potato has protein? Yes, and so do soybeans which have four times the protein of the ordinary beans, avocados, and sunflower seeds, to name a few. This fact, and the high protein in dairy products such as milk and cheese, explain success of vegetarianism. Protein is YOU—it is the material you are made of, from the outer covering of your skin, nails and hair to the hemoglobin flowing in your veins, the hormones affecting your personality, the antibodies, the phagocytes fighting off bacteria and infections and the protoplasm that is the substance of your every cell.

The importance of living on a high protein diet, then, is self-evident. If you are bald, if your teenager totally lacks gracefulness or if you suffer from NERVES, you may be subsisting on a diet which, through the improper combination of amino acids, does not make up a "complete protein". Primarily, the complete protein is to be found in animal sources such as meat, fish, eggs, cheese and poultry. Briefly, amino acids are smaller proteins which have been broken down from gross protein foods. The chopping-up action is performed by yet another group of proteins, the enzymes, as soon as food enters the stomach. Out of approximately 32 different amino acids, the eight most important *must* be eaten in every meal and the others can then be manufactured by the body. This is what is meant by a complete protein. The peanut, for instance, is a great source of protein but lacks one of the eight basic amino acids, which, however, is provided by the whole wheat grain; a peanut butter sandwich, therefore, comprises a complete protein. But, were one to eat the bread first and the peanut butter an hour later, any benefits would be nullified. It is interesting here to note that sunflower seeds are a 'complete-protein' source and that half a cup of these contributes more valuable protein (35g.) than a five-ounce steak (30g.) since muscle meats have a lesser quantity of each of the eight essential amino acids.

Proteins are especially required at breakfast time. This is not an old-wives' tale but a well-authenticated medical fact. Energy is directly related to the blood-sugar level. If this is low, the body does not get enough glucose for fuel; and a condition called hypoglycemia may result.Many a tired, dragged-down-and-out housewife suffers from it.

Carbohydrates

Our main source of energy are the sugars and starches called carbohydrates, which the body breaks down into a simple sugar called glucose. The carbohydrates serve a most necessary function, IF they are derived from a rich, *natural* good source. That excludes the processed and refined starvation-foods which can only be described as deficient, diluted, devoid of good, and dead. The processed white sugar and flour do raise the blood sugar level in the blood momentarily, even though the food is totally lacking in the nutrition the body needs: protein, vitamins, minerals and fats. The result is chaos: the brain receives the message that food (in the form of carbohydrates) has been received, although it does not yet know that this is deficient, poor-quality food. Therefore, it signals the pancreas to release insulin to cope with the sudden influx of sugar, a substance which, unlike protein and fats, is assimilated by the body almost immediately. The hunger pangs are now satisfied, but hundreds of cells are actually dying of malnutrition. This is what happens: insulin, as any diabetic knows, controls the amount of sugar in your blood. If the blood sugar level is low, the liver and the muscles are called upon to release their store of a converted sugar called glycogen; if it is high, the sugar is withdrawn by an extra squirt of insulin. Concentrated sugar, whether from the teaspoon, a candy-bar, a piece of pie, jam or a soft drink, floods the blood with glucose which causes extra insulin to be produced. This results in too much sugar being removed, which leaves you feeling dizzy, tired, irritable and weak. However, had you received your sugar slowly from such foods as meats, milk, fruits (an orange is 10% sugar, a banana 20%), or vegetables (a sweet potato or cooked brown rice is 15%), or unsaturated fats, the digestive process would have introduced the sugar into your system gradually, and you would have received health-sustaining proteins, vitamins and minerals at the same time. A cup of coffee and a doughnut or chocolate bar, then, are the worst food you could eat when you feel low in energy. They bring the blood-sugar level up for an hour without "feeding" you. The slower-acting sugars in proteins, fruits and vegetables, on the other hand, give you a feeling of well-being and energy for five or six hours. This is what makes a well-balanced breakfast of orange juice, bacon, two eggs (protein), toast (preferably whole-wheat), honey and coffee almost mandatory. Any excuse of not being able to swallow a bite for breakfast can be quickly smothered by an edict of an early supper and no desserts, such as ice-cream, to ruin the appetite for the morning. To have a big protein meal at night is utterly nonsensical. What do you want all that energy for at 6:00 p.m.—to help you pick up peanuts (more protein) and the beer bottle while you watch TV? However, if you simply cannot "stomach" the thought of a big breakfast under any circumstances, do read a book by George Watson, Ph.D. called Nutrition And Your Mind (publ. by Harper and Row) who has found that different people have different reactions to different foods. You may be different.

Balance: vitamins, minerals, proteins and carbohydrates are all needed

Vitamins, proteins and carbohydrates are only three of the five basic food elements which keep our body well and functioning at top efficiency. With our modern medicine becoming gradually preventative (at least in North America and Europe) rather than curative, proper nutrition is of considerably greater importance than before.

It is ironic that our dairy cattle, for instance, are fed with much greater care than many of our children. They are given a balanced supplement of calcium, phosphorus, vitamins (A, D), protein in the form of a soya bean preparation, and minerals such as iron, cobalt, iodine, and manganese.

A vitamin deficiency diagnosed early could prevent a serious disease. For instance, fascinating work is being done in Saskatchewan by Dr. Hoffer on the use of Vit. B_3 (niacin) for early treatment in schizophrenia, with an astounding cure-rate.

A close but neglected cousin of the vitamin, however, is the mineral and the two should really be mentioned in one breath. The vitamins in an avocado, for instance, could not work nearly as well, were it not for the preparatory body-building work done by the amino acids and the minerals. Comparable to B-vitamin deficiency is a wide-spread calcium deficiency. This is hard to understand, when we need so much of it for our teeth and bones and since calcium can be found, in milk, yoghurt, cheese, bone meal and greens. The stunted, bow-legged, enlarged-head bodies of post-war children reflected a calcium and vitamin D need. My father, a doctor in Germany after the war, observed a unique solution to the problem which demonstrates how really intelligent our body is and how wise we would be in following instinct or cravings. Tiny babies, less than a year old, would scrape their little fingernails over the calked walls of their brick homes and then contentedly suck on them: it often was their only source of calcium. But how did they know? One of the earlier symptoms of a calcium deficiency is depression or a suffering of "nerves". The need for calcium is increased before menstruation and before puberty—an excellent explanation for premenstrual tension, irritability and cramps. Calcium is also very important in relaxing the heart muscle to slow down the heartbeat. But what should be of great interest and concern to all mothers is that chocolate (as a drink or in candy form) prevents the absorption of calcium into the system at a time when children need it so badly. Carob powder is a delicious substitute that children accept readily. Phosphorus, iodine, sodium, magnesium and many other elements work hand in hand, helping to keep the chain of processes from food to health on-going. Iodine may help to explain the phenomenon of the slender person who can eat anything without gaining weight, chlorine acts as a cleanser, magnesium is a nerve relaxer, and so on. All these elements, however, can be found in our daily food, if it is the nourishing kind: fresh, natural and unrefined. The other mineral that rivals calcium in importance and in which we are often just as deficient is iron. Most people only know that women need it more than men and that its lack can cause a tired, lifeless look and feeling. Iron plays a large part in delivering oxygen to the cells, to keep you from becoming anemic. All weight-conscious readers should perk up here when they hear that by the simple act of adding iron to their diet they can drop pounds. There is no excuse for an iron deficiency—molasses, liver and wheat germ are an excellent source and, if necessary, pills are readily available. For rich, red blood, iron, sufficient hydrochloric acid (which is also needed for dissolving calcium and phosphorus), protein and iodine, folic acid (raw, leafy greens) and the B-complex are necessary.

Vitamins, Oils and Fats

Little by little we are becoming better informed of the vital role balanced nutrition plays. Vitamins, minerals and proteins cause little controversy; carbohydrates, however, are largely misunderstood and fats and oils are actually rejected. Yet these last are our most concentrated forms of energy. Odd as it may seem, they keep our complexions clear, help us to lose weight and actually keep the blood-cholesterol level down. This, however, is only true of the unsaturated fatty acid food products such as vegetable oils (except coconut oil). Of the two types of fats—saturated and unsaturated—our body needs only the latter. Products such as butter, lard, pasteurized milk and, cream, and meat and poultry fats contain both kinds of fat. Solid fats which, to preserve them longer have been irresponsibly hydrogenated, processed cheese and lard are saturated fats and considered no-no's by the experts. This is because they raise the level of cholesterol in the blood-stream. This effect, and a hardening of the arteries by calcium deposits, causes the dreaded artherosclerosis of heart disease. However, it is of interest that eggs fried in saturated (hydrogenated) fats or butter cause a high cholesterol level whereas eggs fried in unsaturated oils do not raise its level at all. Eggs have been much maligned for cholesterol content, but it is less known that they also contain lecithin which is a cholesterol-dissolving agent. Hydrogenation (solidifying liquid fats) is a process similar to the refining of flour for preservation, and it is actually harmful because it robs fat-soluble vitamins of their protection on their journey through the digestive tract. It also upsets proper digestion. When you go shopping for the most healthful oils check the label for the words "pure" and "cold-pressed", since the heating of the oil to keep it from going rancid destroys many vitamins.

Other good fat sources are mayonnaise, nuts and avocados. If you are an economical person, you have probably been guilty, now and then, of eating rancid fats in the form of peanuts, bacon chips fried in rancid fat, walnuts and wheatgerm. Rancidity destroys Vit. E, which in turn influences Vit. A, D and K. It is a well-known sign of the truly good cook that most of his cooking is done on low heat. This is especially true of the fats—they should never smoke, or the irritating acrolein is formed. A third cautioning about fats concerns mineral oil which, since it kidnaps vitamins, should never be used as a laxative, for cooking or even for cosmetic purposes such as baby oil is often used for. To close a discussion of fats a brief mention of lecithin is necessary. It is found in kidneys, brain, egg yolks and soy beans and highly recommended for sufferers from high blood pressure or some coronary diseases. It is a fat that helps to keep skin problem-free, especially in cases of eczema in babies; it protects the nerves, keeps us from getting edgy and keeps the arteries elastic, the liver healthy. You can find it in granular form in most health food stores. Fats and protein are digested more slowly than sugar and are hunger-satisfying and filling for the dieter. If fatty acids are not plentiful enough, food is changed into sugar more quickly and since many "fatties" are really only collecting water, a tablespoon or two of salad oil a day is one way to look trim and fit. My own favourite salad dressing is made of one lemon, a little salt and pepper, some honey and lots of safflower oil, or with the miraculous pure apple cider vinegar, which also has weight-reducing properties.

Vitamin pills: Should anyone take them?

Since I am by no means a nutritionist myself I have faithfully studied the experts and have tried to condense their fascinating and erudite facts on nutrition for brief and easy reading. However, I cannot emphasize enough the importance of reading all of these books yourself at leisure since I have only touched the surface where they have delved. Personally, I marvel at their intimate and diverse knowledge of all the body processes and I devour all new information. Certainly my family is healthier and many complaints have disappeared. Let me stress here that you must not feel guilty if you have been happily misguided in the past or if you do not pop every vitamin into everyone's mouth all the time. Try to organize your findings and then proceed to the best of your ability and according to the availability of products. The body is a miracle and it has managed its smooth functioning for aeons. It is the ill-informed humans with their preserving, processing and polluting who cause disruption and deficiency. If there is a problem, correct it with the proper vitamins and change your eating and living habits generally. It is of course much better to correct a vitamin A deficiency with lots of carrots, apricots, etc. than to pop pills. A bosom loses its tone when it is continually supported by a bra—the muscles should have to do their own work to stay in condition. So it is with the body. It should be encouraged to do its own, age-old work. If we supply the vitamins always through pills the body will begin to rely on them and stop its own vitamin production. Having more or less made up my deficiencies I only take extra vitamins whenever I feel a need for them. When you make up a deficiency be sure to buy the products that are concentrated from natural sources, rather than the synthetic, isolated vitamins sold in many drugstores. Some of these have been found to cause an itchy rash, for instance, as has the eating of white flour products which have been "enriched" with synthetic vitamins. Following is a list of vitamins, their sources, and deficiency symptoms. It would be a wise mother who tacks the list up in her kitchen and checks the symptoms of vitamin deficiency once a month. Then she can set out to correct the problem, for a while, by flooding the menu with natural food sources which are rich in the missing vitamin. Since a *little* knowledge is often a dangerous thing, I would strongly advise you to seek professional help from nutritionists and doctors as you embark on a new health program. Bear in mind also that flavoured vitamin pills are not candies for children and that the principle of "if one is good, ten are better" does not apply to pills of any kind. We are what we eat—a miserable garbage disposal or a blooming fertile field. Perhaps the most dramatic example of my own improvement in health due to nutrition is the never-before-experienced ability to rise up as early as 6:30 a.m. just raring to go. How I used to love my bed, waking up without energy! Now—a stretch, the bounce out of bed, the Abdominal Lift, a shower and the preparation of a big, nutritious breakfast rich in protein and citrus fruit, all follow joyously. My husband couldn't be more delighted.

DAILY REQUIREMENTS

For the greatest amount of energy and bouncing good health you should be eating certain food groups every day. Preferably they should be as close to their natural food states as possible. However, it is quite safe to assume that you are deficient at this moment and should increase your dosage accordingly. It is practically impossible to do harm to your system by overdosing it with vitamins, unless it is in the Vit. B-complex where the vitamins should be taken as a group, not as individual ones. But please remember that vitamins and minerals are brothers and sisters and need each other for greater efficiency and benefit. Everyday, every member of the family should be partaking of all these foods.

1. Fresh fruit at least twice a day, either whole or consisting of one or two glasses of fresh fruit juice, made by you in a blender.
2. Fresh salads made of leafy green vegetables three times a day.
3. Fresh vegetables, barely-cooked or raw at least once a day. Do not ignore such delicacies as tomato, cucumber or bean salad.
4. Fresh vegetable juice, eight to twelve oz.
5. Half a cup of fresh sprouts which you've made yourself from soya or mung beans, rye, wheat, peas, alfalfa, mustard seed, etc.
6. Yogurt—one cup or more, or sour milk, buttermilk and powdered skim milk, milk.
7. An egg, cottage cheese or two to four oz. of unpasteurized cheeses.
8. One or two servings of 100% whole wheat bread, preferably enriched with wheat germ, rice polishings and bran.
9. One serving of meat, fish, soybeans or nuts.
10. Liver, kidney, heart, brain or bone marrow once or twice a week.
11. Iodine—supplied by sea salt, iodized table salt, and ocean foods.
12. Vitamin D—by either sunbathing every day or taking cod-liver oil.
13. And all the "Miracle Foods" listed next.

MIRACLE FOODS THAT SHOULD BECOME A DAILY MUST

To round out your daily diet do become familiar with these easily obtained "extra" foods, which in concentrated, natural form make your search for good family nutrition a breeze. Certainly I try to keep my family supplied with them every day and have noticed a rosy perking up of cheeks, boundless energy and illness-free month after month.

Apple Cider Vinegar—Apple Cider Vinegar acts as a specific for weight-control, bleeding (has a beneficial blood clotting effect and therefore prevents hemorrhages with operations such as tonsillectomies), offsets food poisoning, diarrhea, helps to ease the pain of arthritis, sore throat, laryngitis, acts as a soporific with insomnia, helps with asthma, vertigo, etc. (see the booklet CIDER VINEGAR by Cyril Scott—Athene Publ. Co. Ltd., London).

Almonds—there is some evidence that a substance called laetril in almonds acts as a cancer-preventing agent.(see Edgar Cayce books)

Brewer's yeast—one to two tablespoons in fruit juices or warm water with meals. If a B-vit. deficiency is suspected this dosage can be stepped up to 3 times that amount a day. It is quite palatable and soluble in flake form, undetectable in meat loaf, stews, cereal, etc. Your very deficiency will express itself by gas at first, until corrected.

Calcium—In the form of bone meal, molasses, milk, cheese, soybeans and leafy green vegetables, kelp or dolomite (especially if lacking in hydrochloric acid).

Desiccated Liver—As a revitalizing and cancer preventing agent available in pill form.

Fats—one-two tbs. of pure, cold-pressed salad oil consisting of all vegetable oils, peanut oil or olive oil; butter, cream, fish-liver oils, egg yolk, milk, avocado, animal and fish fats, nuts.

Iron—(and copper) in liver, molasses, wheatgerm, whole wheat, peanuts, apricots, green leaves or "natural" pill form.

Lecithin—especially if there is a record of heart disease or high cholesterol. The phosphorus of protein foods, and fats help to form it. Keeps skin and nerves young and healthy. Found in heart, kidney, brain, egg yolk, and soybeans and lecithin granules.

Molasses (unsulphured)—one to two teaspoons in milk, muffins, cookies, etc. for iron, calcium, sleep cocktail or laxative. Is available in powdered form in health food stores.

Non-instant Powdered skim milk—available in health food stores—looks like cornstarch. Excellent because of low-fat, high protein, high calcium and Vit. B^2 content. Enriches milk, puddings, meat loaves, mashed potatoes, sauces, waffles, muffins, yogurt, without increasing much in caloric content.

Sprouts—If you were on a desert island and were given the choice of only one food to eat for the rest of your life, you would be well advised to choose sprouts. They come from the "seeds of life" and have all the potential energy and food stored for the growing plant. A sprouter is an excellent investment. Use sprouts in salads (potato, spinach, etc.) on their own with dressing, in soups, etc. You can sprout alfalfa, beans, mustard seed, lentil, sunflower seeds, buck-wheat, etc.

Wheat germ and/or Wheat germ oil—the former enriches all baked goods and is considered the best cereal because of B-vitamins, protein and iron and Vit. E content. Should be kept in refrigerator and can be sprinkled on cereals or added to blender drinks.

Yogurt—homemade yogurt has twice the calcium and protein content of the store bought one. Generally speaking Yogurt is also high in riboflavin, but primarily is a wonder food because it is so highly digestible, even to people who cannot tolerate milk. It is an excellent "snack" food when the irresistible urge hits and can be served plain, with lemon-juice and honey, with applesauce, crushed pineapple, grated fresh apple or any fresh fruits to make it palatable for the reluctant.

NATURE'S REMEDIES

NATURAL LAXATIVES

Rarely does one see in its natural state an animal that is constipated, swollen with edema, near a nervous breakdown, bald or arthritic. The delicate balance in nature assures natural medicines and correctives. Since laxatives, particularly the mineral ones, have a tendency to rid the system not only of its wastes but also of the vitamins A, D, E and K as they proceed through the body, they are really a form of poison. Continuous use of laxatives can cause constipation by driving the muscles of the anus to flaccid exhaustion. There are also indications that hepatitis may result. Nature's laxatives provide nutrition while gently encouraging regular bowel movements. Combined with such Yoga exercises as the Abdominal Lift and the Inverted poses, they should bring instant results.

The first two are delicious in warm milk before bedtime and they act as a soporific (sleep-producing) potion as well:

Dark molasses, honey, yogurt, brewer's yeast, wheat germ, apple cider vinegar in buttermilk or combined with honey in water, lots of liquids, milk, herb teas, bananas.

NATURAL DIURETICS

As we become better educated, we hear such terms as diuretics, edema, etc. Women who are overweight hope that it is merely water, which would be easily got rid of. Pregnant women suffer from toxemia. All these terms are connected with the problem of water-retention, for which another name could be urine-storing. This is, of course, a medical phenomenon and must have a cause. It is this very cause that should be corrected, not the end result. Simply to rid the system of water with diuretics (water-releasing pills), does not solve the problem permanently. It does, however, aggravate it in the long run. Water combined with sodium passes into the cells in the first place because a *lack* of potassium has permitted this. Such a deficiency is caused by poor daily diet, too much sugar intake, diuretics and medications like cortisone.

Natural diuretics are: potassium chloride, vegetable oils (linoleic acid), a "complete protein" diet, containing the eight basic amino acids, iron, Vit. B6—taken in natural foods or the B-Vit. compound, and peanuts.

NATURAL TRANQUILIZERS:

If you suffer from "*nerves*", the reasons can also be traced to vitamin and mineral deficiencies. Lack of calcium is the big villain here. But phosphorus (protein foods), Vitamin F (unsaturated fatty acids) Vit. D (sunshine), and phosphatase (enzymes) are all needed for its absorption. However, results will be greatly enhanced by using the Alternate Nostril Breath and other suggested Yoga postures.

Some important natural relaxers are:
Magnesium, the B-Vit. complex, particularly B1, B2 and B6, lecithin, calcium, phosphorus, Vit. F, Vit. D, and Phosphatase.

NATURAL HAIR RESTORERS:

Yoga has exercises for constipation, for nerves, for arthritis and the scalp. But these conditions can be immensely helped by proper nutrition. For the scalp, check this list of goodies to see if *grey hair* or *baldness* can be traced to a lack of these: "complete protein" foods, the B-vitamin inositol, the B-complex vitamins (PABA, biotin, folic acid, pantothenic acid), Vit. E, A & D, calcium, a diet high in protein, cherries, melons, comb honey, raw cream, diets of all-fresh green raw vegetables, bee-venom (through injection).

TIDBITS

Tidbits are brief summaries taken from nutrition books and magazines such as LET'S LIVE and PREVENTION.

NUTRITION

1. For purposes of deriving Vitamin A from carrots, it is better to juice or partially boil them. Only 1% of the carotene from raw carrots is absorbed whereas 5-19% is absorbed from cooked ones.

2. The best source of nutritionally rich sugar is honey, molasses, dried fruit and fresh fruit. Demerara sugar, though better than white, is little more than refined sugar with some molasses added.

3. Your body can receive as much as the equivalent of two cups of sugar from the meats, vegetables, fruits and breads consumed during a day of "sugarless" eating.

4. For a beautiful skin you must use oil from within as well as from without. One or two tablespoons of unsaturated salad oil a day is excellent.

5. The cholesterol level is increased by smoking, alcohol, sugar, carbohydrates and butter (this can be offset by drinking buttermilk, which contains lecithin, in the same meal).

6. Vegetables left uncovered till they wilt and milk which stands in the sunlight lose over 50% of their nutritional value in the first hour. Apples, pears and peaches lose up to 90% if over-cooked.

7. Since many vitamins are water soluble, a great percentage of them is lost by washing slowly, by soaking and boiling or by peeling; exposure to the air destroys the nutrient value.

8. The outer leaves of cabbage and lettuce are up to five times as nutritious as the inner ones.

9. Linoleic acid (in vegetable oils) has been found to relieve eczema and psoriasis because it stimulates the intestinal bacteria that produce the B-vitamins.

10. A peanut butter sandwich (made with unsalted, unhydrogenated vegetable oils) has three times the protein content of a hotdog, a recent study indicated.

11. The sugary creampuff is two to five times more fattening than the starchy hamburger bun, though they are equal in caloric content.

NATURE'S CONTROLS

1. To keep down the salt intake, season eggs and tomatoes with freshly-ground pepper or try fresh lemon juice or nutmeg on many cooked vegetables.

2. Vitamin C is destroyed by smoking. One cigarette destroys the equivalent of one orange.

3. Pulse taking can help you judge if you've had too much sun. If the pulse is two beats higher than before sunbathing, it's time to quit.

4. "Aging may be the result of multiple deficiency states, rather than just 'natural' causes".

5. The high acidic content of citric fruit and its juices and the stickiness of molasses can cause tooth decay. Rhubarb juice can offset their action.

6. Dr. Harry Morrow-Brown, an allergies specialist in England, says not to force children to eat foods they strenuously resist; they instinctively know these may bring on asthmatic attacks.

COOKING METHODS

1. Do all the cooking of vegetables with the lotus-shaped French steamer in the pot to retain vitamins otherwise lost (e.g., Vit. C). Acquaint yourself with the Chinese Wok.

2. Do not force great quantities of new "health-foods" on children. Start gradually with a *bit* of wheat germ on cereal, brewer's yeast and wheat germ in meatloaf, etc. Increase doses slowly and call it natural rather than good or bad food.

HEALTH PROBLEM SOLUTIONS

1. Use one teaspoon pure inositol (B-vit.) in a glass of fortified milk for prevention of baldness.

2. Citric fruit juices are not advised for arthritis sufferers.

3. Potassium chloride is effective in the treatment of hypoglycema (low blood sugar).

4. For a sore, cracked or bleeding anus due to constipation, try inserting a peeled and oiled garlic clove and leaving it over-night.

5. If you suffer from stomach gas it could very well be due to hasty swallowing. Try taking all your liquids through a straw for a while.

6. A person who bruises easily is in need of vitamins C and D.

7. Dr. S. L. Hammar of the University of Washington says that feeding babies solid foods too soon may lead to a life-long weight problem, since the fat cell production takes place at a faster rate in infancy and childhood.

8. Lack of regular dental care and the drainage of poisons from untreated infections in the mouth and throat can be the cause of a multitude of ills, such as arthritis. It is especially dangerous to children suffering of heart ailments, says Dr. Khanna of the University of British Columbia.

FACTS TO PONDER

1. Mother's milk is 250% richer in iron than cow's milk.

2. Dr. J. Yudkin shows a distinct connection between sugar eating and arterial heart disease. People with these complaints have taken up to 100% more sugar than the average healthy person.

3. There seems to be a definite connection between coffee and gray hair and baldness, owing to the deficiency of the B vitamin it causes.

4. Deodorant toilet soaps and after shave lotion may be a factor in allergy to the sun.

5. European studies have linked smoking with decreased sexual activity.

6. There are indications, say researchers at Loma Linda University, that nutritionally-inadequate diets lead to the drinking of more alcohol—as shown by experiments with rats.

7. Non-smokers suffer less from the effect of alcohol than smokers.

8. Cadmium, a harmful chemical in cigarettes, is distributed thus: 6% is inhaled by the smoker, 44% remains in the ash and filter and 50% is distributed in the air for others to breathe. Anyone who smokes more than 20 cigarettes a day suffers as much from impaired vision and judgement as the cocktail-drinker.

B-COMPLEX VITAMINS

SOURCE: Since the B-Vitamins are a complex, that is, they are synergistic, they should not be isolated but given in a common food source. Following is a list of the most common B-Vitamin sources:

Brewer's yeast, liver (and extract), wheat germ and grain, heart, kidneys, blackstrap molasses, rice polishings, brain, muscle meats, egg yolk, whole grains, beans, peas, honey, mushrooms.

Speaking of all the B-Vitamins at once, here are some facts you should know:

1. Antibiotics destroy these vitamins, so that the need for them is increased when on such medication.

2. Yogurt promotes the growth of these vitamins in the intestinal tract.

3. Since they are water soluble, don't discard the cooking water; use it in soups, drinks, etc.

4. First deficiency symptoms occur on the tongue. It should not be coated with visible tastebuds, nor too smooth around the edges. There should be no fissures, no beefy, big tongue look, nor a brilliantly red hue.

Niacin (B^3)—"courage-vitamin", effective in symptoms of pellagra, "nerves", depression, schizophrenia, loss of appetite, diarrhea, insomnia, poor digestion (lack of hydrochloric acid)

Pyridoxene (B⁶)—nerve-relaxer, anti-stress vitamin, effective in trembling palsy (Parkinson's disease), nausea and water retention in pregnancy, migraine headache, excessively oily skin, air and cobalt sickness, expecially effective with magnesium.

Deficiency symptoms: bad breath, irritability, headaches, "nerves", pain and cramps in abdomen, bad-smelling gas, rash around genitals, hemorrhoids, diarrhea, vomiting, dandruff, sore lips and mouth, eczema on face and scalp, dry hands, insomnia.

Pantothenic Acid—"anti-stress vitamin", especially when antibiotics are taken, with burns and severe injuries, effective for burning feet, for grey hair, and wrinkled skin; since sugar or fat cannot be changed into energy without it, people on a diet should make sure of it, also to prevent arthritis and gout.

Deficiency symptoms: hypoglycemia, headaches, dizziness depression, gas, constipation, asthma, stomach ulcers, allergies, insomnia.

PABA—for the prevention of grey hair, mental depression, and needed for conception.

Inositol—effective with baldness and colour of hair, indigestion, hardening of the arteries (because it reduces cholesterol).

Source: Lecithin (heart, kidneys, brain, egg yolk, soybeans).

Choline—"young arteries vitamin" which influences longevity, effective for shortness of breath and heart pain, cirrhosis of the liver, stomach ulcer, muscular dystrophy. A deficiency has been found to cause cancer in animals.

Source: Lecithin.

Biotin—"mental-health-vitamin".

Deficiency symptoms: dry, scaly skin and scalp (eczema), grey skin, nausea, heart pains, depression; in animals, stunted growth and cancer.

Folic Acid—effective in large-cell anemia (can help to gain weight). Deficiency symptoms: fatigue, paleness, dizziness, depression, shortness of breath; very important during pregnancy.

B¹²—fatigue, sore mouth, neuritis, menstrual disturbance, walking difficulties.

YOGA NUTRITION

CALCIUM COCKTAIL STRENGTH-RESTORER FOR MEN (Indra Devi)

Put 8 raw eggs into a jar without breaking their shells. (The eggs should be fertile and must come from chickens that are allowed to run free. Commercially distributed eggs lack certain vitamins.) Cover with the juice of about 16 lemons, preferably grown organically without any poisonous spray on them, and keep in refrigerator for 4-6 days, until shells are dissolved by the lemon and reduced to powder. Take out the eggs, being careful not to break the thin membrane, separate the yolks from the whites, which are not to be used, and put the yolks back into the bowl. Press the contents through a sieve or put into a liquefier, add raw honey to taste and pour in 3-4 ounces of brandy. Keep in refrigerator. Take a tablespoonful 3 times a day before meals, shaking well before using.

CAROB CHOCOLATE MILK SHAKE (Eve Diskin)

4 c. milk
1-3 tbsp. molasses
½ c. non-instant powered milk
⅓ c. carob powder
1 ripe banana
¼ c. nuts
1-3 tbsp. flaked brewer's yeast
1-2 tbsp. wheat germ

Mix in blender and serve.
Start graduating the amount of such strong flavours as molasses, yeast and wheat germ slowly to avoid immediate rejection.

CARROT CAKE

1½ cups Safflower salad oil—cold pressed
2 cups raw sugar.
4 eggs

Mix salad oil and sugar. Then add eggs one at a time and mix after each.
2 cups unbleached white pastry flour or whole wheat flour (fine).
2 tsp. baking soda (sifted then measured)
2 tsp. baking powder
2 tsp. cinnamon
1 tsp. salt
3 cups shredded carrot
1 cup chopped nuts

Sift the above dry ingredients together and slowly add the wet mixture, mixing well. Then add the carrots and nuts, mix, and pour into 3 separate pans. Bake at 300 degrees for 50 minutes or until done.

Frosting can be of your own choice; however, a cream cheese frosting, made from a basic 7-minute double-boiler one with the cream cheese added after cooling, is delicious.

YOGURT (Adelle Davis)

2 cups tepid water
1½ cups non-instant powdered skim milk
Yogurt culture or 3 tablespoons commercial or previously made yogurt

Pour mixture into a pitcher containing:
1 quart tepid water
1 large can evaporated milk

Stir well and pour into drinking glasses or pint jars. Set glasses or jars in dry yogurt maker. If yogurt maker is not used, put into large pan of warm water, bring water level to rim of glasses or jars. Cover pan, and set over pilot light or in warming oven where a temperature of 100 to 120 degrees F. can be maintained. For smaller amounts, heat the milk slightly, then pour mixture into a thermos bottle.

Check consistency at end of 3 hours. Chill immediately after the milk thickens. Yogurt will keep in the refrigerator for 5 days or longer.

Variations:
Serve with brown sugar and cinnamon, honey and finely shredded orange or lemon rind, or sweetened berries, peaches, other fresh fruit or canned applesauce or pineapple.

FRUIT SALAD (Kareen Zebroff)

Make a delicious fruit salad with any fruits you have handy, such as:
2 apples, unpeeled and cut up
½ fresh pineapple, cut up
3 bananas, sliced
2 oranges, sliced or chopped
½ cantaloupe, cut up
1 bunch of grapes
½ c. chopped dates

Add: ⅓ c. liquid honey
1 tsp. cinnamon
½ c. sunflower seeds
1 lemon, juiced

Toss and serve with yogurt.

PEGGIE'S CASSEROLE (Peggie Gabbott)

About 2 cups of pre-cooked Soy beans, Garbonzo beans, lentils or brown rice.
Put into a small casserole.

Make a "Peggy Special", a mixture which can be used in many dishes.

In a wok saute 2 large green onions chopped small.
2 inches of celery.
Green pepper and red pepper if available (makes a nice colour)
About a dozen mushrooms sliced.
About ¼ cup of pine nuts or raw cashews.

Add this mixture to the casserole. Season with a little vegetable salt, and thyme or marjoram or rosemary if liked.
Add 1 cup tomato juice.
Add 1 well-beaten egg.
Mix well and cover with grated mild natural cheese, and sliced tomato if you like. Cover casserole.
Bake until firm at 350 degrees. Uncover for last 10 to 15 minutes to brown cheese and make top crisp.

This is a most versatile casserole. It can be made with any of the above-named legumes. It is delicious when made with curry powder or paste, and about a teaspoon of garam masala, cumin seeds, coriander seads, chopped apple, coconut and raisins.

LIVER CASSEROLE (Adelle Davis)

3 chopped, unpeeled cooking apples
1 chopped, large onion
¾ tsp. salt
½ tsp. freshly-ground pepper
1 lb. sliced baby beef, pork or veal liver
4 slices of bacon cut in half
paprika to taste
¼ c. water or wine

Mix first ingredients well.
Place liver in an oiled casserole.
Cover with apple mixture.
Top this with bacon and paprika.
Add the wine.
Cook in 350° oven for 20-30 minutes.
(For lots of delicious liver recipes, see Adelle Davis' "LET'S COOK IT RIGHT".)

RECYCLED VEGETABLE SOUP (Kareen Zebroff)

4 c. basic broth made from left-over chicken or turkey bones
    Any vegetable water left over from vegetables cooked within the last 24 hours.
2 tbsp. grated carrot
2 tbsp. finely chopped celery
2 tbsp. chopped broccoli
2 tbsp. chopped cauliflower
and any vegetables you happen to have in the fridge such as tomatoes, green peppers, mushrooms, etc.
1 c. of cut-up, roasted old bread
1-2 tbsp. parmesan cheese.

Heat the broth and left-over vegetable water to boiling point.
Add vegetables and let them boil up once.
Remove from heat, add some bread to each soup bowl, sprinkle cheese on top and serve.

BIRCHER APPLE MUESLI

Simply soak overnight one level tablespoon of whole cereal, such as rolled oats, in two tablespoons of water. Next morning, add the juice of half a lemon and one tablespoon of condensed milk, and mix. Quickly shred one large unpeeled apple into the mixture, and stir in a tablespoon each of honey and wheat germ. Serve at once. To increase the protein content you may also add a tablespoon of chopped walnuts, almonds, or sunflower seeds.

SPINACH SALAD (Kareen Zebroff)

1 lb. young spinach
1 handful bean sprouts
3 tbsp. mustard sprouts

Onion Dressing
2 tsp. grated onion
1 tsp. sea salt
½ tsp. freshly-ground pepper
2 tbsp. apple-cider vinegar
8 tbsp. cold-pressed safflower oil
½ tsp. lemon juice

Wash and dry the spinach thoroughly, then chill it.
Mix the first four ingredients of the dressing, then slowly beat in the oil with a
fork till the mixture has the consistency of mayonnaise.
Stir in the lemon juice and pour over the spinach.
Add sprouts just before serving.
Variations: add bacon bits, croutons or strips of fresh chilled fennel.
Optional: Three hard-boiled eggs for garnishing, orange sections.

SUKIYAKI (Kareen Zebroff)

1 lb. flank steak—cut up into very thin slices
⅓-½ cup soya sauce
½ cup hot chicken bouillion (from one cube)
3 tbsp. brown sugar
1 clove garlic, chopped
1 dried ginger root piece—grated

Combine liquids in a flat dish and add sliced meat. Marinate for at least ½
hour, preferably overnight.

1 green pepper, sliced
½ small head of cauliflower
1-2 stalks of broccoli
3 stalks of celery
2 large onions, sliced
3 carrots sliced thinly in rounds
½ lb. mushrooms, sliced or halved
and any vegetable you care to add.

Heat 2 tbsp. of cold-pressed safflower oil to medium heat in a wok and add the
meat to brown. Let the moisture drip off the slices first, but save marinade. Stir
constantly for five minutes. Add marinade and vegetables, cover and cook over
low heat for seven to ten minutes or till vegetables are crisply tender. Serve over
wholewheat noodles or brown rice.

MENTAL HEALTH DRINK (Catharyn Elwood)

1 c. milk (certified, raw, if possible)
1 whole egg
½ fresh, ripe banana
½-1 tsp. carobpowder

  or
1 c. milk
1 whole egg
1 tsp. flaked brewer's yeast
1 tbsp. molasses
½ banana (if desired)

Lack of the B-vitamin biotin can cause mental depression that leads to mild panic. It also causes dry skin, gray complexion, lack of appetite, nausea, pains in the muscles, and disturbance in the heart area. These two drinks and the Carob-chocolate shake are excellent for correcting such symptoms.

CRUNCHY GRANOLA.

6 cups rolled oats
1 cup wheat germ
1 cup fine coconut
1 cup sunflower seeds (chopped)
1 cup all bran (optional)
½ cup honey
1 cup oil, butter or margerine
1 teaspoon sea salt
1 tablespoon milk

Heat the last four ingredients and pour over mixture. Bake one hour at 275°. Stir frequently, leave the oven door open, turn off the heat.

HEALTH BREAD (Peggie Gabbott)

3 cups whole wheat flour
2 tablespoons bran
2 tablespoons wheat germ
2 tablespoons well dried bean sprouts cut up (optional)
2 tablespoons rice polishings
2 tablespoons grated cheese
2-3 tablespoons sunflower seeds
½ teaspoon celery seed (optional)
½ teaspoon caraway seed (optional)
½ teaspoon cumin seed (optional)
1 teaspoon vegetable salt (or sea salt)
1 teaspoon baking powder
1 teaspoon baking soda
2 tablespoons nutritional yeast

Mix:
1½ cups buttermilk
1 tbsp. safflower oil (cold pressed)
Add to solids.
Mix, shape like round loaf, make cross, sprinkle with flour, bake 50 minutes at 350° on a cookie sheet.

Variation:
   2 cups whole wheat flour and 1 cup graham flour, or 3 cups graham flour

Fruit Loaf:
   Substitute honey and/or grated lemon or orange rind, and any kind of dried fruit, dates, chopped figs, raisins, soaked apricots, for the spices.

VITAMINS

BENEFITS	DEFICIENCY SYMPTOMS	FOOD SOURCES
A –VISION, SKIN, MUCOUS MEMBRANES, RESISTANCE TO INFECTION, GROWTH AND REPRODUCTION. Soluble in fats and oils, insoluble in water, not affected by heat, but loses activity if exposed to air at any time. Not affected by alkalies.	A –Night blindness and poor vision or sensitivity to light, dry, scaly skin, gallbladder and kidney stones, poor teeth, retarded growth, thinness, coarse or falling-out hair, pneumonia, inflammation of the reproductive organs, diarrhea, apathy and frequent infections and colds.	A –Green-pigment plants, the greener the better. –Yellow vegetables, peaches, persimmons, yams. –Fish liver oil, liver, egg yolks, milk, butter, cream. –Twice as much is needed when the Vit. A. is derived from carotene.
B¹– (Thiamin)–ENERGY, APPETITE, RESISTANCE TO INFECTION, DIGESTION (HYDROCHLORIC ACID). Soluble in water, insoluble in fats and oils, partially destroyed by pasteurization, intake should be increased when carbohydrates are increased.	B¹ –Slow then rapid pulse, short windedness (athletes need more), poor digestion (gas, constipation), craving for sweets, poor appetite, mental depression, anemia, poor sleep.	B¹ –In the seed: wheat germ, rice polishings, cereal grains, nuts, beans, peas, soy beans, lentils, unrefined bread products, liver (raw), heart, kidneys, brewer's yeast, oysters, barley, asparagus, parsley, raw apple, radish, watercress, lemon, grapefruit, celery, cabbage, carrots, pomegranate, coconut, dandelion.
B²– (Riboflavin)–YOUTHFUL SKIN, VITALITY, LONGEVITY. Soluble in water, not affected by air or heat, destroyed by alkalies and sunlight.	B²–Dim vision, bloodshot and inflamed eyes, oily skin, sore cracked mouth, swollen eyelids.	B² –Liver, yeast, (butter) milk, leafy vegetables (outer leaves are five times better), yogurt, glandular meats, dairy products, raw crabmeat, broccoli, mushrooms, oysters, whole wheat flour, soy flour and beans, apple, apricot, carrot, coconut, dandelions, grapefruit, prune, spinach, watercress.

C —"BEAUTY AND YOUTH" vitamin, STRONG TEETH and BONES, RESISTANCE TO INFECTION, QUICK HEALING OF WOUNDS AND BROKEN BONES, SOOTHING AND BENEFICIAL DURING ANY ILLNESS, ANTITOXIC, PREVENTS FATIGUE. Soluble in water, insoluble in oils, not affected by heat except if exposed to oxygen, destroyed by pasteurization and cooking, but preserved by steaming, somewhat affected by alkalies.	C —Pyorrhea (bleeding, sore gums), scurvy (wrinkles), easy bruising, hives, hay fever and skin infections, feelings of weakness, tender joints, inflamed and infected eyes and cataracts, shortness of breath, headache.	C —Sprouted seeds, young growing plants, apples, oranges, papayas, persimmons, fresh pineapple, rose hips, (green) Puerto Rican cherry juice, bean sprouts, broccoli (leaf), collards, kale, parsley, green peppers, guavas, lamb's quarters, cucumber, grapefruit, rhubarb, spinach, tomato, cabbage, asparagus, carrot, radish, strawberries, bananas.
D —(Other names of artificially produced D2 Vit. ergosterol, viosterol (calciferol), dehydrocholesterol) ENERGY, TOOTH & BONE FORMATION, NERVE-RELAXER. Insoluble in water, soluble in fats and oils, not affected by air or alkalies.	D —Buck and crowded teeth, knock knees, pigeon chest, rickets, "soft" bones, cramps and muscle twitching, fatigue, "nerves", near sightedness, arthritis, loss of calcium in the system.	D —Is the catalyst of calcium, so that the whole calcium family should be taken as well, if deficiencies exist: calcium, phosphorus, Vit. D. and F. iodine, phosphatase. SUNLIGHT is the best source (do not shower for 5-6 hours after exposure), sunlamps in rainy weather, COD LIVER and other fish liver oils, egg yolks and milk (better in the summer).
E —(Alpha-tocopherol)—REPRODUCTION AND SUCCESSFUL PREGNANCIES, GLANDULAR HEALTH, HORMONE PRODUCTION, MUSCLE PERFORMANCE, ANTITOXIC, CARDIO-VASCULAR SYSTEM, GOOD FIGURE (pelvis & bust), PREVENTS THROMBOSIS IN LEGS. Insoluble in water, soluble in oils, not affected by light or heat, destroyed by chlorine.	E —Miscarriage, sterility, muscle degeneration and inflammation, lumbago, bursitis, rheumatism, heart attacks, has been helpful in phlebitis, gastric ulcers, muscular distrophy, multiple sclerosis, menstrual problems.	E —Fresh wheat germ oil, most vegetable oils, fresh cod-liver oils, sardines, shark-liver oil, barley, oatmeal, rye, yellow corn-meal, 100% whole wheat bread, brown rice, butter, eggs, cheese, fish, soybeans, navy beans, kale, parsley, yeast, sweet potatoes, brussels sprouts, leeks, carrots, turnip greens, spinach, watercress, celery, lettuce, apples, bananas, beef liver, kidneys, brain.

MINERALS

Without the proper mineral balance in our bodies we cannot survive. More attention is given to vitamins but many minerals are absolutely essential. I read with interest that doctors fortified the astronauts' diet with potassium to avoid minor heart problems. The following minerals are the most important.

BENEFITS	DEFICIENCY SYMPTOMS	FOOD SOURCES
CALCIUM: Is needed for Vit. D absorption, helps in blood-clotting, promotes regular function of heart muscle, nerve-relaxer, teeth and bone formation. Calcium is especially effective if the Vit. B complex, phosphorus, Vit. D, unsaturated fatty acids, iodine and phosphates are present in the diet.	Poor teeth, stunted growth, "nerves", muscle-spasms, convulsions, cramps, nail-biting, debility, rapid heartbeat, buck teeth, etc.	Milk, leafy greens such as beet greens, broccoli, Swiss chard, kale, collards, watercress, dandelion green, lettuce, spinach, blackberry, cabbage, carrot, celery, cranberry, figs, grapefruit, lemon, orange, rhubarb, parsley, turnip, mustard greens, beans, soybean flour, molasses, bone meal, almonds, cheese, barley-water.
CHLORINE: Is needed for hair growth, body-cleansing and by the digestive juices. It keeps joints flexible and helps in fat-reducing.	In animals: loss of hair, slow growth, apprehension and fear.	Raw meat, salt, milk, legumes, tomatoes, radishes, beets, ripe olives are all good sources.
COPPER: Is needed for the utilization of iron to prevent anemia.	Weakness and poor respiration.	Molasses, liver, oysters, clams, egg yolk, dried fruits (apricots), leafy vegetables, fresh fruit, soy flour, whole wheat grains and loganberries.
IRON: Is needed by every cell for oxygen supply; rosy complexion, vitality; resistance to infection. Chlorophyl is essential in the diet for adequate utilization of iron.	Anemia, fatigue, a gray, wrinkled face, dull hair, flat, cracked fingernails, a sore tongue and mouth and shortness of breath.	Uncooked leafy greens, liver, brewer's yeast, wheat germ, blackstrap molasses, peanuts, all fresh fruits, particularly apricots, soybeans, egg yolks, parsley, tongue, Swiss chard, clams, heart, kidneys, spinach, dates, whole wheat flour, beet greens, beans, bean sprouts, watercress, cabbage, tomatoes, turnips.

Mineral	Deficiency Symptoms	Food Sources
IODINE: Is needed for the smooth functioning of the thyroid gland which is the weight regulator of the body.	Sluggishness, overweight, goiter.	It is found in all seafoods such as cod, haddock, cod-liver oil, oysters, sardines, kelp, dulse, lettuce, potatoes, asparagus, cabbage, carrots, cranberry, cucumber, pineapple, prune, radish, spinach, tomato, watercress, apple, orange, sea salt on foods.
MAGNESIUM: Is especially needed for nerve-relaxation (in conjunction with calcium for depression), and muscle work. It strengthens bones and teeth, and has cholesterol dissolving properties, which in turn dissolve kidney and gallstones. It is also successfully used in treatment of coronary disease, polio, and epilepsy, and helps to prevent constipation, upset tummy and poor circulation.		Nuts (almonds, cashews, peanuts), milk, egg yolk, whole wheat, legumes, lima beans, brown rice, spinach, dates, raisins, grapefruit and orange.
PHOSPHORUS: is the brother to Calcium and is needed to harden and strengthen bones and teeth, is in every cell but is especially prevalent in the brain and sex cells, keeps hair, nails and skin healthy, maintains the alkalinity of bloodstream, helps to form lecithin.	Poor teeth, poor appetite, weight loss, rickets, stunted growth, feeling of weakness.	Protein foods such as meats, milk, eggs, cheese, peas, nuts, soybeans, beans, legumes and all whole grains. For better utilization the diet should also be adequate in hydrochloric acid (B-vitamin complex, specifically thiamin), Vit. D, unsaturated fatty acid and phosphatose.
POTASSIUM: Is needed to balance the supply of food to and disposal of wastes from the cells.	Constipation, "nerves" in the form of insomnia, slow heartbeat, damaged heart muscles and kidneys, infant diarrhea, edema.	Most fruits and vegetables (potatoes) are good sources as are black molasses, almonds and figs, watermelon, bananas, prunes, olives, milk.
SODIUM: Is needed to control the acid-alkaline balance of the blood, keeps calcium in solution and aids potassium in its function.	Retarded and slow growth and underweight, heart-stroke, etc. Too much, however, causes hypertension and water-retention.	Muscle meats and most vegetables. It is better to derive it from natural sources and sea salt than table salt. Whole wheat grains, breads, cheese, buttermilk, spinach, watercress, celery, beets, lettuce and bananas are good sources.
SULPHUR: Is needed to promote the beauty of hair, skin and nails, it has a cleansing effect on the blood and affects body-resistance and liver absorption of minerals.		It is found in some proteins, milk, cheese, eggs, nuts, cabbage, Brussels sprouts, cereals and most fruits and vegetables.

SELECTED READING LIST ON NUTRITION

Title	Author	Publisher
Feel Like a Million	Catharyn Elwood	Simon & Schuster, Richmond Hill, Ont.
Health Through Nutrition	Leford Kordel	MB, N.Y., N.Y.
Let's Eat Right to Keep Fit, and others Let's Cook It Right	Adelle Davis	Signet, The New American Library, Inc. New York.
The Poisons in your Food	William Longgood	Pyramid Publications Inc. New York
Stay Young Longer	Linda Clark	Pyramid Publications, Inc. New York.
A Treasury of Secrets, and others	Gaylord Hauser	Fawcett World Library, New York.
Your Key to Good Health	Carlton Fredricks	London Press, N. Hollywood, Calif.
Eat, Drink and Be Healthy	Agnes Toms	Pyramid Publications, Inc. New York.
Ten Talents	Frank & Rosalie Hurd	Dr. F. Y. Hurd, Box 86A - Route 1, Chisholm, Minn. 55719
The Natural Foods Cookbook	Beatrice Trudy Hunter	Pyramid Publications, Inc., New York.
The Yogi Cook Book	Yogi Vithaldas & Susan Roberts	Pyramid Publications, Inc., New York.
Recipes for a Small Planet	Ellen B. Ewald	Ballantine Books, N.Y.
The Low Blood Sugar Cookbook	Francyne Davis	Grosset & Dunlap, New York, N.Y.

SELECTED READING LIST
FOR HATHA YOGA

Title	Author	Type	Publisher
The ABC of Yoga	Kareen Zebroff	Soft cover	Fforbez Enterprises Ltd., Box 35340,
Yoga for Happier Children	Kareen & Peter Zebroff	Soft cover	Vancouver, B.C.
The Complete Illustrated book of Yoga	Swami Vishnudevananda	Hard cover	Bell Publishing Co. Ltd., N.Y.
Diet, Sex & Yoga	Marcia Moore & Mark Douglas	Hard cover	Arcane Publications, York, Maine, U.S.A.
Executive Yoga	Archie J. Bahm	A "Paperback" Book	Paperback Library Inc., N.Y.
Yoga for Americans	Indra Devi	A "Signet" Book	The New American Library, Inc., N.Y.
Light On Yoga	B.K.S. Iyengar	Hard cover	George Allen Ruskin House London, England.
Rejuvenation Through Yoga	Goldie Lipson	A "Pyramid" Book	Pyramid Publications, Ltd., N.Y.
Yoga and You	James Hewitt	A "Pyramid" Book	Pyramid Publications, Ltd., N.Y.
Yoga for Beauty & Health	Eugene Rawls & Eve Diskin	A "Paperback" Book	Paperback Library Inc., N.Y.
Yoga for Physical Fitness	Richard L. Hittleman	A "Paperback" Book	Paperback Library Inc., N.Y.
Yoga Over Forty	Michael Volin & Nancy Phelan	A "Sphere" Book	Sphere Books Ltd., London, England.

SELECTED READING LIST

MEDITATION

Title	Author	Type	Publisher
Discipleship in The New Age	Alice A. Bailey	Hardcover	Lucis Publishing
The Gospel of Sri Ramakrishna	Ramakrishna Vivekananda Centre	Hardcover	Arcane Publications, York, Maine, USA.
The Yogas and Other Works	Ramakrishna Vivekananda Centre	Hardcover	Arcane Publications, York, Maine, USA.
Yoga, A Scientific Evaluation	Kovoor T. Behanan	Hardcover	Dover Publications, Inc., New York, N.
Yoga, Science of the Self	Marcia Moore	Hardcover	Arcane Publications, York, Maine, USA.
Yoga and You	James Hewitt	Softcover	Pyramid Publication Ltd., N.Y.
Fundamentals of Yoga	Rammurti Mishra, M.D.	Paperback	Lancer Books Inc., New York, N.Y.
Yoga	Ernest Wood	Paperback	Penguin Books, England.
The Autobigraphy of a Yogi	Paramahansa Yogananda	Hardcover	Self-Realization Fellowship, 3880 Sa Rafael Ave., L.A. 65, USA.

EXERCISES in THE ABC OF YOGA

Since this book deals primarily with advanced Yoga poses, I have not always duplicated basic ones. These, however, can be found in the beginners' volume, "THE ABC OF YOGA". Following is a list of its contents.

1. Abdominal Lift
2. Alternate Leg Stretch
3. Ankle Bends
4. Arm and Leg Stretch
5. Arm Lift
6. Blade
7. Boat (Locust)
8. Bow
9. Camel
10. Cat Stretch
11. Chest Expander
12. Cobra
13. Cross Beam
14. Curling Leaf
15. Elbow exercise
16. Eye Exercises
17. Fish
18. Flower
19. Foward Bend (sitting)
20. Forward Bend (standing)
21. Fountain
22. Hands-to-Wall
23. Headstand-Walk Up
24. Japanese Sitting Position
25. Knee and Thigh Stretch
26. Leg-Over
27. Lion
28. Mountain
29. Neck Rolls
30. Pelvic Stretch
31. Pendulum
32. Perfect Posture
33. Plough
34. Posture Clasp
35. Pump
36. Rock 'n Rolls
37. Scalp Exercise
38. Shoulderstand
39. Sitting Warrior
40. Sit-Up
41. Sponge
42. Spread Leg Stretch
43. Toe Exercise
44. Toe Twist
45. Tree
46. Triangle Posture
47. Twist
48. Alternate Nostril Breath
49. The Cleansing Breath
50. Complete Breath
51. Cooling Breath

INDEX